# ACUPUNCTURE

## AN ANATOMICAL APPROACH

# ACUPUNCTURE

## AN ANATOMICAL APPROACH

### HOUCHI DUNG, PH.D.
*The University of Texas Health Science Center,
San Antonio, TX*

### CURTIS P. CLOGSTON, M.D.
*Occupational Medicine, San Marcos, TX*

### JOEMING W. DUNN, M.D.
*Medical Acupuncture, San Antonio, TX*

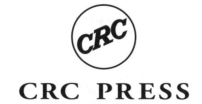

# CRC PRESS

Boca Raton   London   New York   Washington, D.C.

## Library of Congress Cataloging-in-Publication Data

Dung, H. C.
    Acupuncture : an anatomical approach / Houchi Dung, Curtis P. Clogston, and Joeming
W. Dunn.
        p.   cm.
    Includes bibliographical references and index.
    ISBN 0-8493-1651-0 (alk. paper)
    1. Acupuncture. 2. Human anatomy. 3. Neuroanatomy. I. Clogston, Curtis P. II. Dunn,
Joeming W. III. Title.

RM184.D857 2004
615.8'92—dc22                                                                                          2003069581

**Visit the CRC Press Web site at www.crcpress.com**

# Dedication

---

*To our families, in appreciation of their patience and support:*

*Elizabeth Izu Dung*
*Kim B., Curtis and Georgia Clogston*
*Marijo M. Clogston*
*Teresa Lynne, Ashley and Camerin Dunn*
*Y. Ben and Rebecca Dunn*

# Contents

# Acknowledgments

## PHOTOGRAPHY

Photographer: Dennis Havel Photography, Houston, Texas
Models:    Georgia Parker Clogston
    Paul Mills Cooper, P.T.
    Tara Hardcastle
    Lewis W. Koster
    Cathy Rios, M.A.
    George Rios
    Lenora Riser

## CONSULTANTS, MENTORS, SUPPORTERS, STUDENTS

John J. Adams, M.D.
Ann B. Adrian, M.D.
Rhonda Anderson, M.D.
Virgil A. Balint, M.D.
Philip Bamberger, M.D.
D. Paul Barney, M.D.
Marvin S. Belasco, M.D.
Anuthehp Benja-Athon, M.D.
Edward Bennett, M.A., L.N.F.A.
Stacy John Berckes, M.D.
Stephen D. Blood, M.D.
Tamara Boettcher
Larry B. Bragg, M.D.
Paul P. Bricknell, M.D.
Todd Buchanan, M.D.
Ralph L. Buller, M.D.
Lawrence F. Buxton, M.D.
Peter M. Carney, M.D.
Robert J. Casanas, M.D.
Jill A. Castro, M.D.
Ola Gail Caverly, M.D.
Ron Chadiak, M.D.
Pamela Ann Chandler, M.D.
Stanley Chang, M.D.
Linda S. Cheek, M.D.
Boon Y. Chew, M.D.
Jeanne Chiang, M.D.
Brent K. Childers, M.D.
Dennis A. Chu, M.D.
Kenneth Ciolli, M.D.
Albert H. Cobb, Jr., M.D.
Timothy Colt, M.D, J.D.
Mary L. Corbitt, M.D.
Donald Counts, M.D.
Tim Curran, M.D.
Muhammad Dawood, M.D.

Aurora P. De La Rosa, M.D.
Christina de la Torres, M.D.
Carlo Greg Demandante, M.D.
W. John Diamond, M.D.
David L. Diehl
Alan H. Dinesman, M.D.
David Dixon, M.D.
A. Lynn Dolson, M.D.
Mary Douthit
Mitchell Elkiss, M.D.
Edwin Falconi, M.D.
Wenlin Fan, M.D.
Lynne Fenton, M.D.
Mitchell Finney, M.D.
Michael Fredericson, M.D.
Gilbert Garcia, M.D.
Michael B. Gluth, M.D.
Mary Ann Gonzales, M.D.
Dave Greenberg, M.D.
Dayton F. Haigney, M.D.
David E. Hallstrand, M.D.
Paul L. Hannah, M.D.
Peter G. Hanson, M.D.
Robert E. Harvey, M.D.
Fred Hilton, M.D.
Jennie S. Huang, M.D.
Jonie H. Huang, M.D.
Leslie Huszar, M.D.
Carl Jenkins, M.D.
Susan Joerns, M.D.
James A. Johnson, M.D.
Mark Johnson, M.D.
David C. Jones, M.D.
Jeffrey W. Jordan, M.D.
Anand Joshi, M.D.
Joseph K. Haddad, M.D.
Gail Scott Honorka, M.D.
Matt Hummell, M.D.
Susan Kallal, M.D.
Hyo S. Kim, M.D.
Sung S. Kim, M.D.
Neil B. Kirschen, M.D.
Johanna S. Koch, M.D.
Tong-Chui Koh, M.D.
Constantine A. Kotsanis, M.D.
Rebecca Kragh, M.D.
Andres Lee, M.D.
Ann Lee, M.D.

Harold Lee, M.D.
Dee Wee Lim, M.D.
Suzanne Lima, M.D.
Diane Linda, M.D.
Frank M. Lobacz, M.D.
Timothy S. Lyda, M.D.
Leonid Macheret, M.D.
Charles R. Massey, M.D.
Joyce Mauk, M.D
Anna C. Miller, M.D.
Robert D. Milne, M.D.
Richard Moczygemba, M.D.
Josue Montanez, M.D.
Bufford Don Moore, M.D.
Greg Moore, M.D.
James W. Moyle, M.D.
Susan Murphey, M.D.
Manuel S. Naron, M.D.
William C. Nemeth, M.D.
Sai H. Oh, M.D.
Melanie Olsen, M.D.
Bruce D. Oran, M.D.
Glenda J. Peters, M.D.
Michael D. Pettibon, M.D.
Thai T. Phan, M.D.
Stuart C. Pipkin, III, M.D.
Stephanie M. Prado, M.D.
Barbara Randolph, R.N.
William H. Rice, M.D.
Tommie M. Richardson, M.D.
Emilia Ripoll, M.D.
Charles H. Ripp, M.D.
Timothy O. Rowe, M.D.
Carmen Rumbaut, L.M.S.W., J.D.
Richard A. Sandler, M.D.
Paul R. Satwicz, M.D.
Roger Moss Saulson, M.D.
Jason Schillerstrom, M.D.

Don R. Schulte, M.D.
Marjorie Shuer, M.D.
Mark K. Smith, M.D.
Rivers Sterling, L.Ac. (NCCAOM)
Donald D. Strobel, M.D.
William J. Tarver, M.D.
Teruko Tashiro, M.D.
Charles H. Tegeler, M.D.
Robert Q. Terrill, M.D.
Gregory M. Thomas, M.D.
Sheri Thomas, M.D.
Alfred S. Tung, M.D.
Bill Uncapher, M.D.
Jorge Villalobos, M.D.
Khai Van Vo, M.D.
Chris Walhberg, M.D.
Bryan K. Walker, M.D.
Jack L. Walzel, M.D.
Ching M. Wang, M.D.
Clifford J. Ward, M.D.
Joseph Wong, M.D.
Brian Woods, M.D.
Jun-Yi Wu, M.D.
Harley W. Yoder, M.D.
Harvey Yung, M.D.
Jeff Zucherman, M.D.

**WEBSITE FOR MORE INFORMATION**

www.anatomicalacupuncture.com.

**E-MAIL**

info@anatomicalacupuncture.com.

**WEBSITE FOR OTHER ACUPUNCTURE RESOURCES**

www.crcpress.com (search on the term "acupuncture").

# Preface

I think it was probably 1999 when Houchi Dung* first called to say he wanted to teach me acupuncture. I had known Dr. Dung for nearly 30 years; he was one of my interviewers when I applied to medical school, and once I was accepted and matriculated, he was one of my teachers of gross anatomy (a subject in which I did not excel). When he called those many years later, he said he was preparing to retire from the university and he wanted to teach me acupuncture. Why me? He did not say at the time, but later he admitted it was because of my journalistic background. He felt a communicator was necessary to convey what he had learned over his 30-year career of sticking some 5 million needles into some 16,000 patients. In fact, he said that the reason he pushed for my acceptance into medical school was because the medical profession needed to be able to communicate better.

I was skeptical. My (uninformed) opinion of acupuncture was that it was placebo, pure and simple. Furthermore, to my thinking, it was based on metaphysical concepts that are incongruent with the principles of medicine. I put Dr. Dung off for nearly a year before he wore me down. For one thing, I had a lot of respect for him, and I owed him a debt for his supporting my medical career at an important time. In retrospect, his persistence was uncanny. He wanted me to spend a week or two at his clinic — he said that would be enough time to learn all I needed to know. I could not spare the time as a block. Reluctantly, he agreed to let me come on Saturday mornings, although he feared that would not give me the needed perspective to learn how to manage patients. I came to his clinic every Saturday morning for over a year, observing his patients and then incorporating what I had learned in the treatment of my own patients.

As I said, I was skeptical. I was hoping to spend a few Saturdays at his clinic and then quietly fade away back to my more pressing duties. Little did I know what was in store for me. First, I had to admit almost immediately that acupuncture is not a placebo; it was obvious that Dr. Dung's patients were helped! Second, there was nothing metaphysical about his teaching. He was the same scientist I had known as a student, and he disdained nonscientific concepts of acupuncture. Dr. Dung had taken classical acupuncture and reinvented it as a medical science. His meticulous observations of his patients (and some 2,000 cadavers) over his career had led to some important discoveries, which he was generously willing to share with any practitioner willing to take the time to learn them.

Dr. Dung has an overriding desire to see acupuncture understood as science and taught, along with gross anatomy, in medical schools throughout the world. He published his first book, *Anatomical Acupuncture*, in 1997; it contains a wealth of knowledge but is somewhat difficult to read. He wanted me to help him write a revised edition of that text, but we ultimately settled on the entirely new text here before you. This current text borrows heavily from the earlier one, with the authors' thanks to its publisher Antarctic Press for allowing us to do so. Dr. Dung has traveled throughout the U.S. and the world to promote the use of acupuncture in medical education, and his earlier book has been translated or is being translated into several languages. Its first printing in Chinese sold out in China, indicating its relevance in a country in which acupuncture is an accepted practice.

Almost immediately after beginning my studies with Dr. Dung, I began incorporating acupuncture into my practice. It was so easy and patients responded so well! It is gratifying in clinical practice to obtain such dramatic results, even in refractory cases, and with so little effort. Dr. Dung is an anatomist as well as an acupuncturist, but not a physician, so his career has been limited in that he cannot diagnose disease and has often been deprived of the benefit of knowing a patient's complete medical history. Some of the case histories in this text reflect that deficit. His son, co-author Joeming Dunn, M.D., is a physician who limits his practice to acupuncture and has taken over his father's practice since his retirement.

I have a more comprehensive practice, seeing acute occupational injuries and offering a variety of therapeutic options other than acupuncture: medication, education, and physical therapy. Many of my patients are blue-collar workers with little sophistication, and it has been difficult to introduce some of them to acupuncture. I rarely do at first, preferring to wait until it has become obvious that they are not progressing with other therapies and may require surgical intervention. (I have had patients waiting interminably for insurance approval for epidural steroid injections by a pain medicine specialist. After I administered acupuncture in the interim to provide symptomatic relief, they refused the epidural injections once approval was finally obtained because by then they were asymptomatic.)

I have had to overcome quite a bit of initial patient resistance, especially in males, because of fear of needles. Employers, too, are resistant, often feeling, as I once did,

---

* Pronounced Dō-ŏng.

that acupuncture is bogus. Gradually, though, the former find acupuncture more palatable than other available options (and are gratified to find that the pain of an acupuncture needle is not at all like that of an injection). The latter are beginning to see that the judicious use of acupuncture saves them money because their employees' recoveries from painful conditions are accelerated without more extensive and expensive interventions. Gradually, I have begun to use acupuncture for sinus allergy and asthma with gratifying results, and I look forward to trying it in a number of other conditions, especially infertility.

I am grateful to Dr. Dung for his helping me to understand more about the subject of pain. This is a greatly overlooked topic in medical education, and he has added new knowledge to the understanding of pain progression throughout an individual's lifetime. This is one of the most important themes of this text — possibly more important than the description of the practice of acupuncture. I am also grateful for his giving me a tool to help so many patients so easily and giving me the opportunity to assist in the production of this text. His selflessness, honesty, and integrity as a person and as a scientist have propelled this project forward, hopefully to the benefit of millions of our readers' patients.

**Curtis P. Clogston, M.D.**

# The Authors

**Houchi Dung, Ph.D.,** a native of Taiwan, earned his Doctor of Philosophy degree in anatomy from the University of Louisville, Kentucky. For nearly four decades, he has taught anatomy and acupuncture, primarily at the University of Texas Health Science Center at San Antonio, Texas, most recently as an Associate Professor in the Department of Cellular and Structural Biology. He has been a member of many academic societies including the Southern Society of Anatomy, the Texas Society for Electron Microscopy, the American Association of Anatomists, the American Society of Zoologists, the Society for Neuroscience, the American Pain Society, the American Society of Clinical Anatomists, the International Society for the Study of Pain, the American Society for Cell Biology, the New York Academy of Science, and the Texas Acupuncturists Association. He has served on the Editorial Board of the American Journal of Chinese Medicine, the National Advisory Board of the National Back Foundation, and the Texas State Board of Acupuncture Examiners. He has written numerous academic publications in the fields of anatomy and acupuncture. His first text, *Anatomical Acupuncture,* has been circulated throughout the world and translated into several languages, including Chinese. Dr. Dung has been a tireless traveler worldwide to educate physicians about the value of incorporating acupuncture into traditional medical practices, especially for pain and respiratory allergy management.

**Curtis P. Clogston, M.D., J.D.,** is a diplomate of the American Board of Preventive Medicine and practices preventive and occupational medicine in San Marcos, Texas. A graduate of the University of Texas Health Science Center at San Antonio, Texas (UTHSCSA), he has been the Medical Director of the City of San Antonio Emergency Medical Services, Allied Health Program Director in EMS at UTHSCSA, and a clinical instructor in Orthopaedics/EMS, also at UTHSCSA, where he was the author of numerous articles and presenter of academic presentations in the field of emergency medicine and emergency medical services. He also graduated with a Doctor of Jurisprudence degree from The University of Texas School of Law and has practiced legal medicine with the Office of the Attorney General of the State of Texas and the Office of the Chief Counsel of the United States Food and Drug Administration in Washington, D.C. Dr. Clogston started a computer enterprise focusing on medical practices and the use of geographic information services (GIS) in healthcare applications. He learned acupuncture in 2000 from Dr. Dung and has incorporated it into his practice, primarily for the management of pain and of allergies affecting the respiratory system.

**Joeming W. Dunn, M.D.,** is a graduate of the University of Texas Medical Branch at Galveston, Texas. He received advanced training at the Presbyterian Hospital in Dallas (Internal Medicine) and the University of Texas Southwestern Medical Center, also in Dallas (Nuclear Medicine). He currently practices anatomical acupuncture in San Antonio.

# 1 Acupuncture and Medicine

## CONTENTS

## 1.1 A BRIEF HISTORY

Acupuncture is a very old practice reputed to have originated in China,[1,2] although some have attributed its origin to Egypt, India, or even Japan.[3] Hippocrates is said to have inserted needles into patients' ears to cure impotence.[4] In 1991, the remains of a man who died approximately 5000 years ago were found in the Alps between Austria and Italy. Ötzi, as his discoverers called him, had 57 acupuncture points tattooed on his body.[5]

The Chinese are known to have practiced acupuncture for approximately 2000 years, although it was nearly forgotten until the Communists resurrected it and forced their Western-style physicians to learn traditional Chinese medicine. The first reported use of acupuncture anesthesia in China (for tooth extractions) was in 1960; it was claimed that 70% of patients experienced no pain with acupuncture anesthesia, 27% had mild pain, and 3% failed to respond.[6] The use of acupuncture anesthesia was then extended to other types of surgery, including appendectomy, meniscus repair in the knees, thyroidectomy, gastrectomy, retinal operation, craniotomy, pulmonary resection, hysterectomy, and open-heart surgery.[7] References to acupuncture in Chinese medical literature disappeared during the Cultural Revolution. However, interest resurfaced in the early 1970s with President Richard Nixon's historic trip to China when acupuncture anesthesia was shown off to many Western journalists and scientists.[8–10] Use of acupuncture anesthesia has since waned in China, mostly because of physicians' inability to predict which patients will benefit from its use and probably also because its efficacy had been greatly overstated.

Today in China, as in much of the Western world, the medical establishment disdains acupuncture as unscientific. In the West, acupuncture is associated with Oriental culture and has heavy metaphysical baggage. Although it has been in practiced in the U.S. for more than 150 years,[11] including in the management of low back pain,[12,13] its use remains controversial.

## 1.2 CURRENT MEDICAL LITERATURE

The confusion about acupuncture in current medical literature reflects the difficulty of studying acupuncture in randomized controlled trials (RCTs). It is hard to blind a subject or investigator as to whether or not the subject is receiving a needle stick. The most frequent method of attempted blinding is to use so-called sham acupuncture, which is the placement of needles in areas that are not on traditional Chinese meridians. It is the contention of the authors of this text that needles stimulate peripheral nerves rather than meridians (which have no anatomical manifestation); almost no place in the human body does not have at least some peripheral nerves, so it is likely that so-called sham acupuncture has at least some therapeutic effect by stimulating the nervous system. Another issue is the selection of subjects: different patients have different results from acupuncture and other treatments (including medication) used to mitigate pain. This text will demonstrate a method of predicting these patients' responses to acupuncture; without distinguishing among them, it is hard to attain statistically significant results in a clinical trial.

Yet another issue is chronicity. This book shows that acupuncture is most effective when used early in the treatment of pain; it is unfortunate that many patients try acupuncture as a "last resort" after wasting months or years with other forms of therapy. Authoritative reviews describe many or most acupuncture trials as poorly controlled or too small to produce significant results. Nevertheless, despite these difficulties, sources (such as *Clinical*

*Evidence, The Cochrane Review,* and *Effective Health Care*) find evidence that acupuncture may be effective in treatment of lateral elbow pain, primary dysmenorrhea, headache, and dental pain, as well as certain nonpainful conditions such as the nausea and vomiting associated with surgery and cancer therapy. The more recent editions (as of this writing in August 2003) of these reviews are summarized in the paragraphs that follow.

Generally, acupuncture is described in *Effective Health Care* as most often used in management of chronic musculoskeletal pain.[14] This citation describes the poor quality and conflicting results of RCTs evaluating the effectiveness of acupuncture. One review finds insufficient evidence about the effectiveness of most physical treatments, including acupuncture, for neck pain.[15] This is not surprising for the reasons described previously. It is not surprising that investigators have difficulty blinding for other physical treatments; it is difficult to imagine the contents of sham massage or sham physical therapy.

In the treatment of back pain, van Tulder and Koes (in *Clinical Evidence*) find two systematic reviews that conclude no significant difference exists between acupuncture and placebo or no treatment in the management of chronic low back pain and sciatica. However, they do find a systematic review and an RCT that conclude that acupuncture is superior to transcutaneous electrical nerve stimulation (TENS) in reducing pain intensity and increasing overall improvement.[16] Van Tulder and another set of reviewers (in *The Cochrane Review*) find that 11 trials of "low methodological quality" do not prove that acupuncture is beneficial in the treatment of low back pain.[17] Again (in *Clinical Evidence*), van Tulder and Koes found no RCTs and no systematic reviews of acupuncture in acute low back pain.[16]

In the treatment of lateral elbow pain, Green et al. find insufficient evidence to support or refute the use of acupuncture, although they find two small trials that indicate a short-term benefit in this condition.[18] Farquhar and Proctor (in *Clinical Evidence*) found that acupuncture is superior to placebo or no treatment in relieving the pain of dysmenorrhea.[19] Melchart et al. (in *The Cochrane Review*) concluded that

> [o]verall, the existing evidence supports the value of acupuncture for the treatment of idiopathic headaches. However, the quality and amount of evidence are not fully convincing. There is an urgent need for well-planned, large-scale studies to assess the effectiveness and cost-effectiveness of acupuncture under real-life conditions.[20]

Goadsby (in *Clinical Evidence*) cites a small RCT that found no evidence that acupuncture is effective "with episodic or chronic tension-type headache, although the trial was too small to exclude a clinically important effect."[21] Zakrzewska (in *Clinical Evidence*) found no evidence

about the effects of acupuncture in the treatment of trigeminal neuralgia.[22] A review in *Effective Health Care* found acupuncture to be effective for post-operative dental pain.[14]

The reader can see that evidence for or against acupuncture in the treatment of pain is quite limited. Research is difficult because of the blinding issue and the lack of an accepted scientific underpinning to the practice — it seems contradictory to base a scientific study on a metaphysical discipline. This text squarely addresses the latter issue, as Dung did in his earlier work, by providing a scientific underpinning to acupuncture. It is hoped that the information presented here will suggest new strategies for coping with the former issue. It seems highly unlikely that people would keep sticking needles into themselves and each other for 5000 years across several continents if it were not effective to do so; the authors' decades of combined experience with acupuncture have found it rewardingly efficacious in treating pain *in selected patients*. They hope that the information presented here will spur further research in this important area.

In conditions other than pain, some evidence supports the efficacy of acupuncture, although the authors of this text are at somewhat of a loss to explain some of the mechanisms of action. The review in *Effective Health Care* cited above supports the use of acupuncture in controlling nocturnal enuresis and postoperative and post-chemotherapy nausea and vomiting, but not in tinnitus, plaque psoriasis, or addictions such as smoking and overeating.[14] Dung occasionally uses acupuncture for tinnitus and smoking cessation, but not for overeating, having long ago found it ineffective; Clogston rarely uses acupuncture for overeating or smoking cessation because of discouraging results with the latter and no experience with the former. The authors find acupuncture effective in treating allergy and asthma in approximately 75% of cases. Dung has used it in treating infertility in women with close to 50% success in the most difficult cases (those who had tried everything else first) and has had some success with treating urinary incontinence in older women.

Acupuncture has virtually no application in conditions affecting motor nerves, as is pointed out in the Appendix. A possible exception is Bell's Palsy, which is discussed in Chapter 11.

## 1.3 AN ANATOMICAL APPROACH

The ensuing chapters and the appendix describe the features of acupoints as neural tissue. They will describe chronic pain as a progressive and largely irreversible condition of the peripheral nervous system. A technique for assessing patients to determine their lifetime experience of pain and to predict their response to therapy will be described; however, these tools are only about 85% accurate, so the reader would be well advised to consider that individuals vary. Additionally, these chapters will discuss and illustrate the technique of acupuncture and, finally, will apply this knowledge to treatment of various conditions, primarily pain, allergy, and asthma. It is expected that this information will help the clinician use acupuncture effectively in his or her practice as a supplement to comprehensive medical care.

The reader is cautioned that, although acupuncture "appears a relatively safe treatment in the hands of suitably qualified practitioners, with serious adverse events being extremely rare,"[14] its inappropriate use can be dangerous, as in the treatment of chest pain, cancer, or even arterial hypertension. In the latter condition, even if acupuncture is effective, its effects are undoubtedly temporary; also, there is significant risk that an overly optimistic patient may discontinue his medication and be lost to follow-up, leading to serious consequences. If the reader is alert to these risks and those associated with needling a few anatomical areas near vital structures, he or she will find acupuncture efficacious, safe, and surprisingly easy to learn, as seen in the chapters that follow.

## 1.4 A BRIEF NOTE ABOUT THE TERM *NEUROMODULATION*

It has been suggested that the concepts in this book and in Dung's previous text have changed acupuncture into something else. That is not entirely true. Although most of the acupoints in this book have equivalents in traditional Chinese medicine, some are different. More importantly, the intellectual underpinning as a medical science is definitely different.

*Neuromodulation* has been suggested as a more appropriate name to apply to acupuncture as described in this text — that is, acupuncture as a technique based on neuroanatomy and physiology to modify the functioning of the nervous system. To distinguish the two, *acupuncture* is defined as an art based on traditional Chinese medicine that involves insertion of fine needles into certain points on the skin for therapeutic purposes; *neuromodulation* is defined as stimulation of the nervous system by whatever means to affect its functioning. As so defined, neuromodulation could include TENS or trigger point injections. The practice of neuromodulation according to this definition falls squarely within the practice of Western medicine. The difference between neuromodulation and traditional Chinese acupuncture carries implications regarding licensing and certification. To avoid cutting too fine a line between the two terms, "acupuncture" will be used throughout this book to represent "neuromodulation" performed with needles, that is, stimulation of the nervous system with needles to affect its functioning.

## REFERENCES

1. Veith, I. Acupuncture in traditional Chinese medicine — an historical review. *Calif. Med.* 118:70, 1973.
2. Veith, I. *The Yellow Emperor's Classic of Internal Medicine*. University of California Press, Berkeley, 1970.
3. Australian Medical Acupuncture Society. History of acupuncture. www.ozacupuncture.com.
4. Lewith, G.T. The history of acupuncture in the West. British Medical Acupuncture Society. www.medical-acupuncture.co.uk.
5. www.discovery.com/exp/humancanvas/humancanvas.html.
6. Sheng, L.C. and Chang, T.H. Electroacupuncture anesthesia in oral surgery — a preliminary report. *Chin. Med. J.* 80:97, 1960
7. Shanghai First People's Hospital. Acupuncture anesthesia in thyroidectomy. *Chin. Med. J.* 2:17, 1973.
8. Diamond, E.G. Medicine in the People's Republic of China — a progress report. *JAMA* 222:1588, 1972.
9. Sidel, V.W. Medical education in the People's Republic of China. *New Physician* 284 (May), 1972.
10. Reston, J. Now about my operation in Peking. In *The New York Times Report from Red China* by Durdin, T., et al. Quadrangle Books, New York, 1971, pp. 304.
11. Lee, W.M. Acupuncture as a remedy for rheumatism. *Boston Med. Surg. J.* 15:85, 1836.
12. Osler, W. *The Principles and Practice of Medicine*, 7th ed. D. Appleton & Co., New York, 1909.
13. Edwards, A.R. *A Treatise on the Principles and Practice of Medicine*. Lea Brothers & Co. 1183, 1907.
14. Acupuncture, *Effective Health Care*, 7(2), 2001. www.york.ac.uk/inst/crd/ehc72.htm.
15. Binder A. Neck pain. *Clin. Evid.*, 2002 June; (7)1049–62.
16. van Tulder, M. and Koes, B. Low back pain and sciatica: chronic. *Clin. Evidence*, June (7), 2002.
17. van Tulder, M.W., Cherking, D.C., Berman, B., Lao, L., and Koes, B.W. Acupuncture for low back pain (Cochrane Methodology Review). In: *The Cochrane Library*, Issue 3, John Wiley & Sons, Ltd., Chichester, UK, 2002.
18. Green, S., Buchbinder, R., Barnsley, L., Hall, S., White, M., Smidt, N., and Assendelft, W. Acupuncture for lateral elbow pain (Cochrane Methodology Review). In: *The Cochrane Library*, Issue 3, John Wiley & Sons, Ltd., Chichester, UK, 2002.
19. Farquhar, C. and Proctor, M. Dysmenorrhea *Clin. Evidence*, June (7), 2002.
20. Melchart, D., Linde, K., Fischer, P., Berman, B., White, A., Vickers, A., and Allais, G. Acupuncture for idiopathic headache. *Cochrane Rev.* (3), 2002.
21. Goadsby, P. Chronic tension-type headache. *Clin. Evidence*, June (7), 2002.
22. Zakrzewska, J. Trigeminal neuralgia. *Clin. Evidence*, June (7), 2002.
23. Bosson, S. and Lyth, N. Nocturnal enuresis. *Clin. Evidence*, June (7), 2002.
24. Thorogood, M., Hillsdon, M., and Summerbell, C. Changing behaviour. *Clin. Evidence*, June (7), 2002.

# 2 Characteristics of Acupoints and Their Significance

## CONTENTS

## 2.1 ACUPUNCTURE, ACUPOINTS, AND TRIGGER POINTS

*Acupuncture* is traditionally defined as the insertion of fine needles into certain points on the skin for therapeutic purposes. A similar term, as defined in the previous chapter, is *neuromodulation* — the stimulation of the nervous system by whatever means to affect its functioning. However, to avoid confusion by making too fine a distinction between these terms, "acupuncture" will be used to encompass both of these concepts; hereafter it will be used to mean *stimulation of the nervous system with needles to affect its functioning.* In acupuncture, needles are inserted into points on the skin called *acupoints* (convenient shorthand for acupuncture points). Although a great deal of controversy surrounds some of the terms used here, the authors believe that acupoints are synonymous with "trigger" points, "motor" points, "tender" points, "sensitive" points, and "derma-" points described by authors and researchers such as Vanderschodt,[1] Melzack,[2] Liu,[3] Bonica,[4] and Travell and Simons.[5]

Acupuncture's primary use is in treatment of pain, acute or chronic. Many other uses, such as treatment for sinus allergy, asthma, and infertility, will be described later in this text. Acupuncture has been promoted by some for uses that defy physiological explanation and should be approached with caution. Also, some applications, such as treatment of hypertension, may be inappropriate. Although it is known that acupuncture can reduce blood pressure, the duration of the effect in each individual patient is unknown, so careful ongoing follow-up is necessary and uneven control can be expected.

## 2.2 ACUPOINTS AS AFFERENT NERVES

Acupoints are loci on the skin that, when stimulated with needles, produce desired physiologic effects. These points overlie afferent (sensory) nerves of the peripheral nervous system or, in a few cases, other richly innervated tissue. These afferent fibers carry general sensation from the periphery of the body to the central nervous system. (It is expected that the reader is a medical professional and has a general understanding of anatomy. The authors have included a brief review of the pertinent neuroanatomy in the Appendix. Also, using a standard anatomy atlas will be quite helpful while reading this text.) Dung has described in an earlier work how, as an associate professor of anatomy at the University of Texas Health Science Center at San Antonio, he participated in the dissection of approximately 2000 cadavers to explore the underlying anatomical structure of 112 mostly classical acupoints selected from traditional Oriental texts.[6] Most of these 112 points are bilateral, with 13 in the midline, resulting in 211 loci on the body. The authors of this text will borrow heavily from Dung's earlier work.

These afferent peripheral nerves have anatomical characteristics that predict their likelihood of forming acupoints; these will be explored later in this chapter. One important property of acupoints is that they change phase under certain conditions.

## 2.3 PHASES OF ACUPOINTS

Acupoints may or may not be tender to about 1 kg (2 to 3 lb) of palpation pressure (which will be referred to as *standard palpation pressure*; if not stated otherwise, any reference to palpating an acupoint means to palpate it with standard palpation pressure), or an acupoint may be a source of pain without any palpation whatsoever. If the point is not tender at all to standard palpation pressure, it is said to be in the *latent phase*. If it is tender to palpation but not actively producing pain, it is said to be in the *passive phase*. If it is producing pain without any palpation pressure, it is said to be in the *active phase*. When a patient can put a finger on the exact location of his or her pain, it is most likely that this active point is one of the 112 acupoints described in this text. These distinctions among phases are quite important and will be referred to throughout this book.

## 2.4 SIGNIFICANCE OF PHASES OF ACUPOINTS IN ASSESSMENT AND TREATMENT

The concept of phase needs to be understood for two important reasons. First, assessment of the proportion of acupoints in the passive phase has prognostic significance; second, to be effective, acupuncture needles should be placed into points that are either passive or active; it is relatively useless to place needles into latent points.

A patient who has a large percentage of points in the passive phase is less likely to benefit from acupuncture treatments for pain. This is typically the patient who cannot get relief from pain using over-the-counter medications and may need to rely on narcotics. The worst of these patients have pain when touched firmly anywhere on the body and are often said to have *fibromyalgia* (a misnomer for a real and debilitating condition). Most likely, these patients may have surgery, for example, for carpal tunnel syndrome or temporomandibular joint syndrome but continue to have pain postoperatively. They are unlikely to get relief with any pain management regimen short of narcotics.

Acupuncture can help some of these patients but the effect, unfortunately, is incomplete and relatively short-lived. It is important to select out these patients so they can be appropriately counseled and referred for other treatment, such as a multidisciplinary pain program. However, it must also be said that some of these patients obtain at least temporary relief from acupuncture; in difficult cases, needles may be the only available option. (Also, it should be kept in mind that the system described here is imperfect; it is accurate in 85% of patients, which implies that almost one-sixth of patients will benefit from acupuncture despite a large number of passive points or fail to benefit despite a small number.) Fortunately, the group of patients with large numbers of passive points constitutes only a small portion of all pain sufferers.

More fortunate patients have only a few acupoints in the passive or active phases; these are the points that will be needled during acupuncture treatment. The results of treating these patients for pain are usually quite good. Before exploring this topic further, it is time to examine another feature of acupoints: they have a fairly predictable sequence of changing from latent to passive — a process that, for simplicity, will be called *conversion*.

## 2.5 CONVERSION OF ACUPOINTS FROM LATENT TO PASSIVE

Acupoints convert from latent to passive in response to pain, which contributes to conversion for *exogenous* and *endogenous* reasons. The exogenous reasons are typically acute injuries suffered primarily in the home, at work, in sports, or in motor vehicle accidents. These are usually *local* (*regional*) in nature, meaning that the injury is confined to a discrete area of the body and that acupoints appear (i.e., become passive or active) only in that discrete area — at least acutely. Initially, only the locus of injury will be tender, but if the injury is severe and protracted enough, other points in the general area of the injury and, ultimately, throughout the body, will become tender as well.

In contrast, endogenous reasons are *internal to the body*. The causes may be focal, resulting from disease of an internal organ (gastric ulcer, for example), or systemic such as diabetes and thyroid disease. It is interesting that focal causes can cause tenderness in acupoints on the skin that share the same dermatome as the internal organ; an example is tenderness of points overlying the xiphoid process of the sternum in patients with gastritis or gastric ulcer disease. The systemic causes are often contributory, in that they do not produce pain but may affect the severity or quality of pain in general. These causes are complex and poorly understood but may indicate direct damage to nerves, as in the insensitivity to peripheral pain often seen in late-stage diabetes.

Whether the cause of pain is exogenous or endogenous, the chronic effect of pain on acupoints is progressive. As a person's lifetime experience of pain increases, more and more points throughout the body become passive in a fairly predictable sequence. The reason for this progression is uncertain, but its effect is as if the entire peripheral nervous system becomes progressively more inflamed in response to accumulated pain. Factors that are poorly understood may speed the progression and others may retard it, but the basic sequence of progression is the same in virtually all individuals. It should also be noted that early in the progression, when few acupoints are passive, it is possible for some of them to revert to the

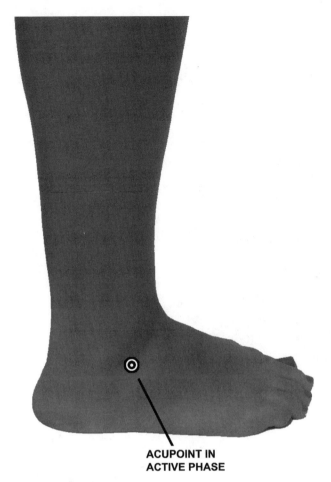

**ACUPOINT IN
ACTIVE PHASE**

**FIGURE 2.1a** The original ankle sprain creates tenderness at the tip of the lateral maleolus due to stretching of the calcaneofibular ligament, which is richly innervated by branches of the sural nerve. The associated acupoint, the Inferolateral Malleolus, immediately converts to the active phase (indicated by a target symbol).

latent phase, but as more and more acupoints become tender, this becomes less likely. It will be seen in the following pages that the conversion of acupoints from latent to passive or active phase can be local in nature, as when an ankle is sprained and the acupoint at the tip of the distal fibula becomes tender, or systemic, when points throughout the body become tender in response to pain anywhere in the body.

An example will show the interplay between local and systemic responses. An injury producing at first local and then systemic conversion is an ankle sprain in a healthy person with little or no lifetime history of painful events. The person will develop an active acupoint at the site of injury (Figure 2.1a) and, within hours or days, a few passive local points around the ankle (Figure 2.1b.). As the injury heals, the local points will become less tender and most will completely disappear, while systemically the individual may develop a few other bilateral pairs of passive points throughout the body (Figure 2.1c). The systemic points become passive in a predictable sequence.

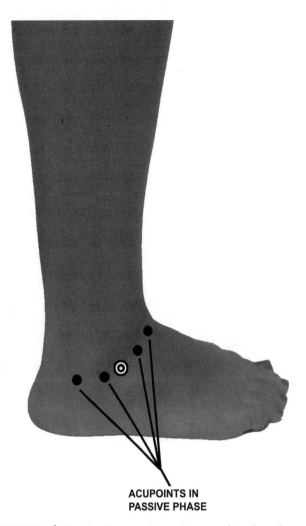

**ACUPOINTS IN
PASSIVE PHASE**

**FIGURE 2.1b** In a few hours or days, other acupoints along the sural nerve become passive, although the Inferolateral Malleolus point may become less tender. The size of the affected area is an indication of the acuteness or chronicity of the pain; a concentrated reaction indicates a more acute injury.

The first of these will most likely be along the deep radial nerves in the forearms near the elbows. The second will be along the great auricular nerves under the ears and the third will be along the spinal accessory nerves on the tops of the shoulders near the neck.

The number of systemic points to convert depends on a number of factors, including the severity and duration of the painful event, the person's age and general health, and possibly psychological factors. If later the same individual experiences another painful episode (e.g., lateral epicondylitis, as shown in Figure 2.1d), more local points will appear and subsequently disappear for the most part while additional, more or less permanent systemic points will appear, again in predictable sequence. (Furthering the example, these would likely be the saphenous nerve just distal to the knee, followed by the deep peroneal nerve in the foot and the tibial nerve in the leg, as shown in Figure 2.1e).

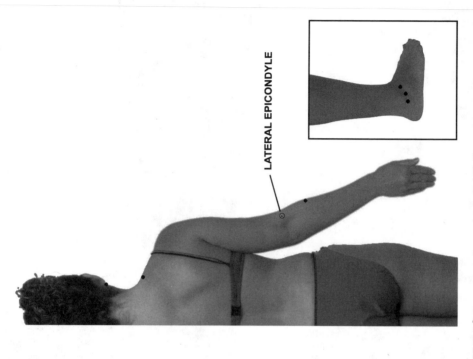

**FIGURE 2.1d** Some time later, the individual sustains another injury, for example, a tennis elbow (lateral epicondylitis), and has a new active acupoint on the lateral epicondyle. Other passive acupoints may appear around the affected elbow.

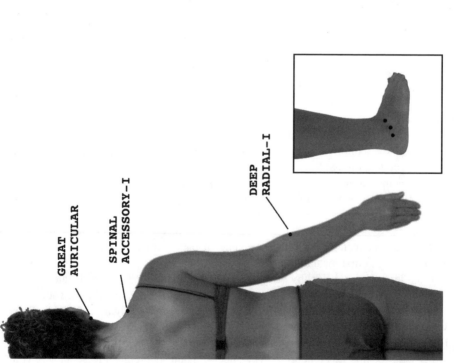

**FIGURE 2.1c** After several weeks, systemic acupoints convert to the passive phase in a predictable sequence: the Deep Radial-I acupoint in the forearm; then the Great Auricular under the ear; and then the Spinal Accessory-I on the top of the shoulder near the neck. As shown in the figure, the local points near the ankle may return to the latent phase and the affected area may shrink, but the systemic points most likely will stay passive throughout the individual's lifetime. Eventually, the original point of injury at the inferolateral malleolus may revert to the latent phase, or it may stay passive indefinitely.

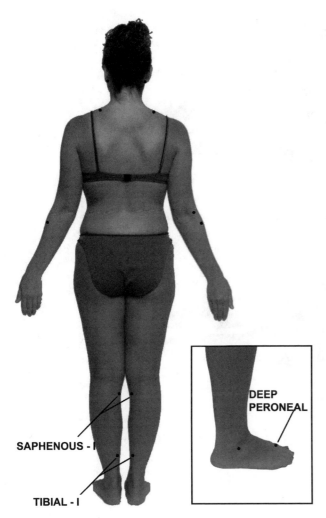

SAPHENOUS - I

TIBIAL - I

DEEP PERONEAL

**FIGURE 2.1e** Later, the tennis elbow has resolved, but the patient is left with more passive systemic acupoints: the Saphenous-I in the leg; then the Deep Peroneal in the foot; and then the Tibial-I in the lower medial leg. If the injury has fully resolved, the lateral epicondyle may be completely latent (in this figure, it is shown as still passive).

Another example is shown in Figure 2.2a and Figure 2.2b, depicting the progression of tender acupoints in a woman with severe menstrual cramping. This condition, dysmenorrhea, can be focal in nature, as in cases of endometriosis or endometrial cysts, but evidence also indicates that it is humoral. During menstruation, acupoints throughout the body, and especially those in the genital region, become more tender to palpation and to acupuncture needles. These humoral effects require more study to determine if they are a result of circulating menstrual hormones acting on the nerves or a result of other hormones that generally mediate all pain responses. Either way, dysmenorrhea is easily the most important source of pain in women.

The authors believe that severe menstrual pain should be aggressively treated because, as the condition goes untreated, more and more systemic acupoints appear

(become passive), possibly leading to a diagnosis of fibromyalgia at the conclusion of a 40-year reproductive life. These individuals experience pain if touched virtually anywhere on the body; thus, it is the authors' hypothesis that fibromyalgia is a disease of the nervous system damaged by excessive exposure to pain. The condition is insidious, in that acupoints become passive gradually but inexorably, in the same sequence to be seen in an individual with exogenous injury, but progressing further through the sequence because of the quantity and intensity of pain. These women often relate a history of being unable to get out of bed during their menstrual periods because of the severity of the pain and tell of undergoing a hysterectomy at an early age. In contrast, a woman without a history of menstrual pain will likely develop far fewer passive acupoints during her life; those that develop will be primarily in response to periods of acute pain associated with illness or injury.

Another interesting point is that the drop-off in concentration of passive acupoints around an exogenous injury, such as the sprained ankle discussed earlier, is indicative of the degree of acuteness or chronicity of the injury. For example, in the healthy person with a history of little lifetime pain who suffers a sprained ankle, an early concentration of local passive acupoints would immediately surround the point of injury. As time passes, more passive points would appear at a distance from the injury. Eventually, most or all of the local points would disappear leaving only a few systemic points distributed throughout the body. It can be seen that the effect of the injury spreads out through the body over time, leading to the conclusion that an acute injury produces points painful to palpation only at the site of injury, to be followed over time by an expanding zone of passive points.

The sequence of the acupoints' conversion is quite useful and is the foundation of the principles of assessment introduced in the next chapter. Specific anatomical features of peripheral nerves determine this sequence.

## 2.6 FEATURES PREDISPOSING ACUPOINTS TO CONVERT TO PASSIVE PHASE

Ten features of peripheral sensory nerves are associated with forming passive acupoints, as described by Dung.[6] Each of these is explored in more detail next:

1. Size of the nerve
2. Depth of the nerve
3. Emergence of the nerve from deep fascia
4. Passage of the nerve through foramina in bone
5. Presence of neuromuscular attachments
6. Presence of concomitant blood vessels
7. Composition of the nerve
8. Presence of nerve bifurcations

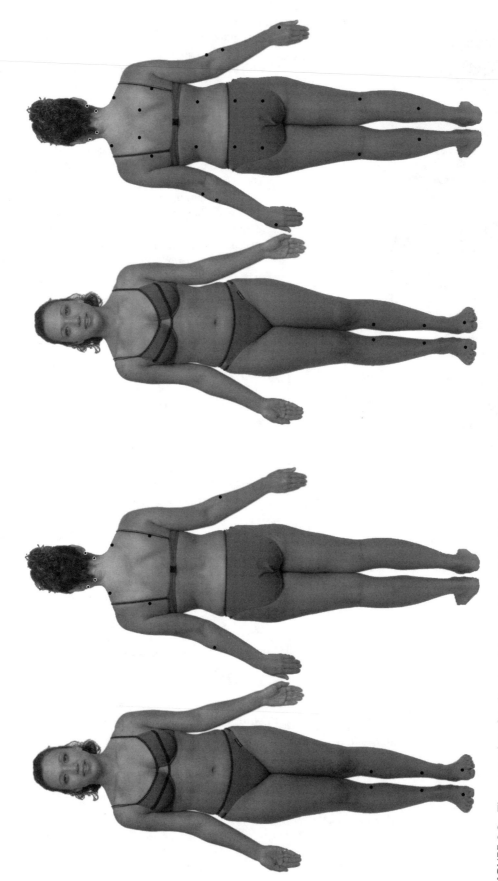

**FIGURE 2.2a** The progression of tender acupoints caused by a lifetime history of severe dysmenorrhea: after five years of untreated dysmenorrhea (assuming no other injury or source of pain), approximately 16 points have become passive (tender).

**FIGURE 2.2b** The progression of tender acupoints caused by a lifetime history of severe dysmenorrhea (continued): after 10 years of untreated dysmenorrhea, approximately 32 points have become passive.

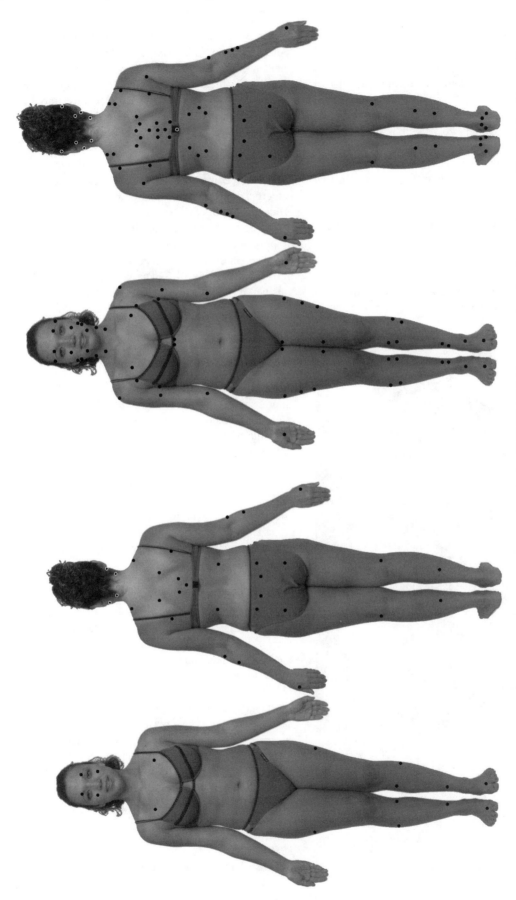

**FIGURE 2.2c.** The progression of tender acupoints caused by a lifetime history of severe dysmenorrhea (continued): after 15 years of untreated dysmenorrhea, approximately 48 points have become passive.

**FIGURE 2.2d.** The progression of tender acupoints caused by a lifetime history of severe dysmenorrhea (continued): as a rule of thumb, each five-year period of untreated dysmenorrhea causes another 16 points to become tender. If a woman has a 40-year history of dysmenorrhea, 128 points will be passive (shown).

9. Association with sensitive ligaments
10. Association with suture lines of the skull

The *size of the nerve* bundle is an important factor affecting the sequence of conversion because larger bundles are more likely to become passive. However, other factors sometimes outweigh size, as will be seen later. An example is the two important acupoints at the elbow formed by two different cutaneous nerves: the lateral antebrachial and the medial antebrachial (Figure 2.3). Each of these two cutaneous nerves becomes superficial at the elbow after coursing more deeply inside the brachium (upper arm), and it is only as they become superficial that they form acupoints. The nerves are essentially similar in all respects except that the lateral one is larger and as a result is a more important acupoint.

The *depth of the nerve bundle* can outweigh size in importance, as in the case of the sciatic nerve in the gluteal

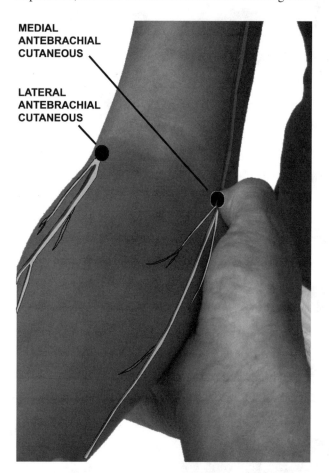

**MEDIAL ANTEBRACHIAL CUTANEOUS**

**LATERAL ANTEBRACHIAL CUTANEOUS**

**FIGURE 2.3** The lateral and medial antebrachial cutaneous nerves form acupoints after they emerge to a superficial level from deep fascia. The examiner's thumb is on the acupoint formed by emergence of the medial brachial cutaneous nerve through the fascia; the lateral brachial cutaneous has a corresponding acupoint as it emerges from the deep fascia of the brachium. The lateral nerve is larger than the medial one and thus forms a more important acupoint.

region, where it is the largest nerve in the body. No acupoints are along this nerve until it becomes more superficial on entering the posterior compartment of the thigh and the popliteal fossa. Proximally, the nerve is deep in the thick gluteus muscles and practically impossible to palpate from the body surface. Similar examples may be found along other nerve trunks. The brachium (upper arm) has relatively few acupoints because nerve bundles in this area are deep in muscle mass or buried inside the neurovascular compartment. Once they emerge to a more superficial location, acupoints are more likely to form. Thus, the depth of the nerve bundle is an important factor in the development of acupoints, although usually not as important as the size of the nerve.

The *emergence of the nerve from deep fascia* is also illustrated in Figure 2.3. The lateral antebrachial cutaneous nerve is seen to be forming its acupoint as it emerges from the deep fascia of the brachium. Other cutaneous nerves also form acupoints as they emerge through deep fascia; the medial brachial cutaneous is another example.

*Passage of nerves through bony foramina* to distribute subcutaneously is seen in the face. The cutaneous branches of the trigeminal nerve in the face, such as supraorbital, infraorbital, mental, zygomaticotemporal, and zygomaticofacial, have acupoints where they penetrate the bony foramina (Figure 2.4a and Figure 2.4b).

*Neuromuscular attachments* are sometimes referred to as *motor points*.[7,8] In this text, the more precise term *neuromuscular attachment* refers to the site where a muscular nerve branch (consisting of motor, sensory, and sympathetic fibers) attaches to and enters a muscle mass. In many gross anatomy texts, a muscle is often illustrated as having numerous neuromuscular attachments from a single nerve trunk. However, at close inspection, it is apparent that a nerve trunk approaches its muscle at a single locus in most cases, unless the muscle is relatively long, in which case two neuromuscular attachments will be present.

Of course, there are as many potential acupoints as there are neuromuscular attachments, but in fact most of these attachments are deep within muscles and thus not likely to become tender to palpation. The best and most obvious example of an acupoint associated with a neuromuscular attachment is the deep radial nerve at the lateral surface of the proximal portion of the forearm between the muscles of the brachioradialis and the extensor carpi radialis longus (Figure 2.5). The deep radial nerve is relatively deep inside the septum of the two muscles at this location, and its associated acupoint where it has several neuromuscular attachments has a greater probability to turn tender than that of the nearby lateral antebrachial cutaneous nerve, which is approximately the same size. In fact, more than 99% of individuals who come to the authors' clinics with pain exhibit tenderness at the deep radial point.

*Concomitant arteries and veins* course with nerve trunks that reach muscle masses at the neuromuscular

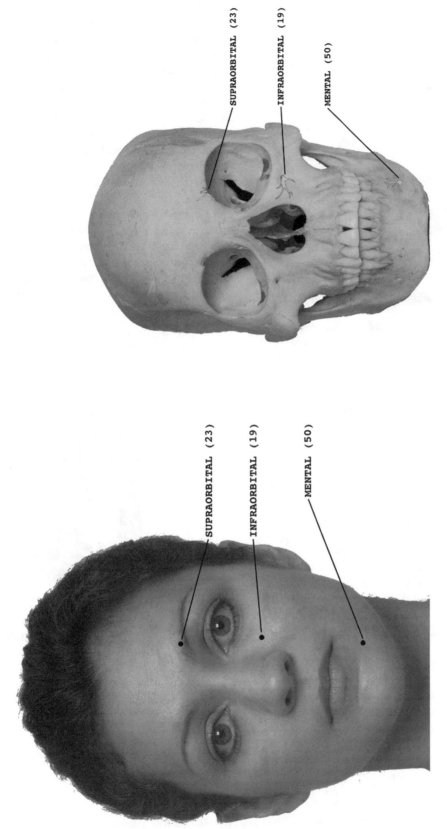

**FIGURE 2.4a** Depicted on a live model: acupoints are formed where nerves emerge through bony foramina in the face.

**FIGURE 2.4b** Depicted on a skull: acupoints are formed where nerves emerge through bony foramina in the face.

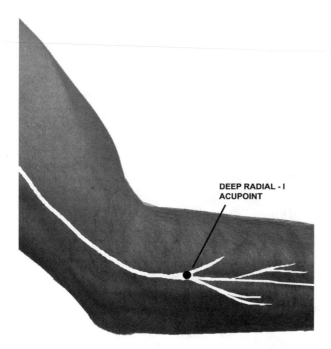

**FIGURE 2.5** Anatomic location of the deep radial nerve and its most prominent acupoint where the nerve bifurcates and makes attachments with the surrounding muscles. Points such as this are sometimes called *motor points*.

attachments. These nerves, arteries, and veins coursing together are often called *neurovascular bundles*. The physiologic role of blood vessels in the formation of acupoints is not known. Nevertheless, blood vessels in the vicinity of neuromuscular attachments often are associated with these points becoming tender at an early stage of pain progression. In contrast, many cutaneous nerves are found without concomitant blood vessels, and even though some of them are superficially located and equivalent in size to branches of the muscular nerves with blood vessels, the points formed by the latter can be far more tender than those formed by the former. One such example is the deep radial nerve and the lateral antebrachial cutaneous nerve discussed in the previous paragraph: the former is associated with blood vessels and the latter less so; this factor and the previous one (neuromuscular attachments) may not be completely independent in that the deep radial nerve example chosen to illustrate this point exhibits both features. Certain cutaneous nerves exhibit this phenomenon too, such as the supraorbital and infraorbital nerves where they emerge through the skull with associated blood vessels. However, this factor is not completely independent from the factor of passage through bony foramina discussed earlier. The interrelationship of these factors shows the difficulty of determining their relative importance.

*Nerve fiber composition* is important in that cutaneous nerve branches have only afferent and postganglionic

sympathetic fibers, while muscular nerve branches have these two types of fibers and also the larger efferent (motor) fibers to skeletal muscle. When all other anatomic features remain the same, acupoints formed by the muscular branches with their three different types of fibers are more likely to become tender than those formed by the less varied cutaneous branches. Therefore, nerve fiber composition constitutes an anatomic *feature* of acupoints (although it may not be a truly independent *factor* for their formation).

*Bifurcation points* are the locations at which nerves divide into smaller branches. Strictly speaking, locations where a peripheral nerve penetrates the deep fascia; passes through a bony foramen; or enters the muscle mass at the neuromuscular attachment are places at which the branching of nerve bundles and trunks occurs. However, nerves bifurcate at other places as well, and these bifurcations can form acupoints. The nerve trunks on which acupoints form in this manner are located in the distal portions of the upper and lower limbs, particularly in the dorsal, palmar, and plantar surfaces of the hand and foot (Figure 2.6).

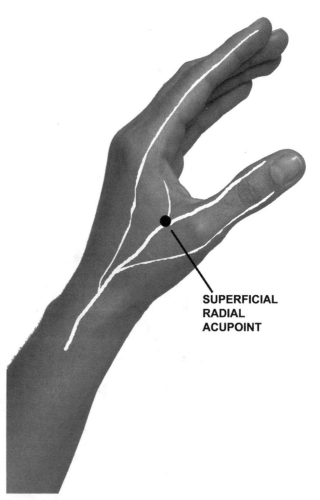

**FIGURE 2.6** Bifurcations of the superficial radial nerve and a prominent acupoint formed at a bifurcation.

*Highly sensitive ligaments* include muscle tendons, bone retinacula, thick fascial sheets, joint capsules, and collateral ligaments formed by dense fibrous connective tissue. These structures are known to contain rich afferent nerve receptors and to be sensitive to pressure, palpation, or stretching. These sensitive loci can also become acupoints. Two examples are the tendons of the biceps brachii muscle lodging in the intertubercle groove of the humeral head (conversion of which to passive phase accompanies biceps tendinitis), and origins of the long extensor muscles of the forearm from the lateral epicondyle of the humerus (associated with tennis elbow). As will be seen in the next chapter, the ligamentum nuchae covering each of the thoracic spinous processes is another example of these sensitive ligaments. Finally, there are acupoints often palpable along the suture lines (i.e., coronal, sagittal, and lambdoidal) of the skull. Patients with chronic headaches develop tenderness at these locations.

The anatomic features reported here are not intended to be inclusive; other anatomic features may contribute to the formation of acupoints. However, the 10 factors or features described earlier help predict the sequence of the appearance of acupoints in individuals with acute or chronic pain. An acupoint demonstrating more of these characteristics is likely to become tender earlier in the progression of pain than one demonstrating fewer of them.

An alternative hypothesis for the predictable sequence of the appearance of passive acupoints is that all peripheral nervous tissue becomes equally sensitive in response to pain and that certain mechanical features of palpating this tissue predict its perceived sensitivity. For example, the nerves emerging from the foramina of the skull have bone directly beneath and relatively little overlying tissue; about 1 kg (2 to 3 lb) of palpating pressure effectively traps these nerves between the palpating finger and bone and creates far more pressure on the nerve than would applying the same pressure on another nerve buried deep within tissue. In the latter case, the surrounding tissue would absorb most of the palpating pressure.

Highly sensitive ligaments demonstrate the same characteristics as the acupoints in the face: they usually are next to bone and close to the surface, facilitating a painful vice-like effect with a small amount of palpating pressure. Adding these mechanical factors to the amount of nervous tissue present under the palpating finger would allow a simpler model to be developed. This model would use only the amount of pain and resulting reactivity of nervous tissue; the amount of tissue, and the effective force applied to the tissue. Clearly, more research needs to be done in this area, but the choice of model is mostly irrelevant from a clinical point of view: the reactivity of passive acupoints to standard palpating pressure is a useful assessment tool, as will be seen in the ensuing chapters.

## 2.7 PAIN QUANTIFICATION USING PASSIVE ACUPOINTS

In the preceding discussion of significance of the phases of acupoints, it was mentioned that the percentage of acupoints in the passive phase has prognostic significance for acupuncture and other interventions. Dung in his previously cited work devised a 12-point *pain quantification* scale, based on the proportion of 112 points* in the passive phase. On that scale, zero indicates that no points are passive and 12 indicates that most or all of them are.

A patient's pain quantification (also called *pain sensitivity* in this text) can be determined by two methods. The first consists of palpating certain of the thoracic spinous processes with a standard palpation pressure and deriving pain sensitivity from the number of processes that are tender. This is a simple method but requires the patient to partially disrobe. The second method is perhaps more clinically useful, but requires specific knowledge of the anatomical location of a significant number of acupoints and their likely sequence of becoming tender. Both methods of quantifying pain will be introduced in the next chapter.

## REFERENCES

1. Vanderschodt, L. Trigger points vs. acupuncture points. *Am. J. Acupuncture* 4:233, 1976.
2. Melzack, R. Myofascial trigger points: relation to acupuncture and mechanisms of pain. *Arch. Phys. Med. Rehabil.* 62:114, 1981.
3. Liu, Y.K. et al. Correspondence between some motor points and acupuncture loci. *Am. J. Chin. Med.* 3:347, 1975.
4. Bonica, J.J. Definitions and taxonomy of pain, in *The Management of Pain*, 2nd ed., Lea & Febiger, Philadelphia, 21, 1990.
5. Travell, J.G. and Simons, D.G. *Myofascial Pain and Dysfunction: the Trigger Point Manual*. Williams & Wilkins, Baltimore, 3, 1983.
6. Dung, H.C. *Anatomical Acupuncture*. Antarctic Press, San Antonio, 1997.
7. Gunn, C.C. and Milbrandt, W.E. Tenderness at motor points. *J. Bone Joint Surg.* 58:815, 1976.
8. *Dorland's Illustrated Medical Dictionary*, 26th ed., W.B. Saunders Corp., Philadelphia, 1978.

* To be exact, Dung used 110 points in his earlier work. The list is slightly revised in this text and the 112 points are extrapolated from Dung's original 110.

# 3 Pain Quantification

## CONTENTS

## 3.1 INTRODUCTION

Pain quantification is the process of determining or estimating the proportion of 211 representative acupuncture points on the body that have converted to the passive phase. These points consist of 99 bilateral points (giving 198 points adding both sides of the body) and 13 midline points (spinous processes of T1, T3, T5, T6, T7, T9, and T10; bregma; nasion; depressor septi; mentalis; sternal angle; and occipital protuberance). The bilateral points are usually equivalent on either side of the body and are considered together. Thus, we will speak of a scale based on 112 acupoints, consisting of 99 points found on either side of the body and 13 points found in the midline. Basically, all bilateral points are counted as single points. (Because a bilateral point is usually passive or latent on both right and left sides of the body, a point on one side is considered to have the same sensitivity as the one on the other; if one is tender, both are assumed to be tender for pain quantification purposes and are not counted twice. If a discrepancy between the two sides occurs, it is usually because of a local injury on the more tender side.)

The major benefit of pain quantification is in estimating an individual's lifetime experience of pain and in predicting his or her response to acupuncture and other pain therapies. This is done by estimating the percentage of these points in the passive or active phases. The direct method is to palpate each of the 112 points and record the patient's responses. Two more practical, indirect methods are to: (1) palpate some of the thoracic spinous processes and (2) palpate representative acupoints on other areas of the body. Easier and less time consuming than the direct method, each of these indirect methods is described in this chapter.

## 3.2 PAIN QUANTIFICATION USING THORACIC SPINOUS PROCESSES (METHOD ONE)

Anatomically, it is known that the tips of the spinous processes are joined by a strong supraspinous ligament that expands to form the ligamentum nuchae in the cervical and thoracic regions. At the attachments of the ligament to the spinous processes, there are numerous free nerve endings — terminals of unmyelinated and finely myelinated afferent fibers presumably mediating pain sensation. It is unknown if one spinous process has more of these free nerve endings than others. However, these processes become tender to standard palpation pressure in a predictable sequence, and the most logical explanation is that they have different quantities of *nociceptors* (nerve receptors for the sensation of pain; see the Appendix for a general discussion of neuroanatomy).

There are 12 thoracic spinous processes, but only 6 of the first 9 are important for this discussion.* The following descriptions of anatomical locations assume that the individual being examined is lying in the prone position with arms at the sides; this position most approximates the anatomical relationships seen in the standing position, shown in Figure 3.1. Also, in this text, the vertebral segments are indicated in the usual manner of using a letter (i.e., "C," "T," or "L") to represent the level of the spine (cervical, thoracic, or lumbar, respectively) and a number to represent the position of the vertebra within that level.

---

* One or two other spinous processes could have been added to this schema by Dung in his earlier work,[1] but they were disregarded, to no apparent detriment. The authors will continue to use Dung's earlier system in this text.

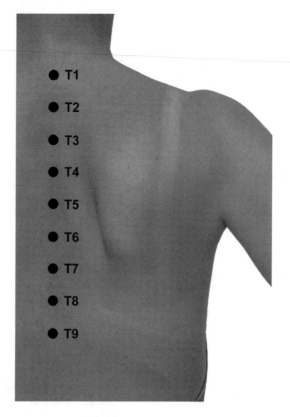

**FIGURE 3.1** The first nine thoracic spinous processes. This model is standing to emphasize the surface anatomy, but a patient is usually examined in the prone position, with arms at the sides of the body, when being assessed using Method One.

The first thoracic (T1) spinous process is located 1 to 2 cm inferior to the prominence of the C7 spinous process. The T3 spinous process is at the level of the bases of the spines of the scapulae. The T7 spinous process is at the level of the inferior angles of the scapulae and in women is often found right above the superior margin of the brassiere strap. The remaining spinous processes are determined by finding T1, T3, or T7 and then palpating and counting adjacent processes.

The system of quantification described next is performed as follows: the patient's back is exposed with the patient in the prone position. The spinous process of T7 is identified and standard palpation pressure, typically with the tip of the thumb or index finger, is applied to it. The patient is queried as to the presence of tenderness and its extent and the response is recorded. This is repeated for T6 and T5 but T4 is skipped. The process is repeated for T3 and T1, omitting T2. The process is finally repeated for T9, for a total of six spinous processes.

Once the responses have been recorded, they are scored with two points allocated for spinous processes on the upper extreme of tenderness and one point for those that are only mildly tender. No points are allocated for nontender processes. The points are summed, with the

result expected to lie on a scale from 0 to 12. The resulting number is one estimate of the individual's pain sensitivity. (For example, if T7 and T5 are tender, T3 is mildly tender, and the rest are nontender; compute by adding two points for T7 plus two points for T5 plus one point for T3, giving five points total and indicating a pain sensitivity of five on a 12-point scale.)

## 3.3  DISCUSSION OF METHOD ONE OF DETERMINING PAIN SENSITIVITY AND THE SIGNIFICANCE OF PAIN LEVELS

The six acupoints used in this method have long been known to traditional acupuncturists but the significance of their sequence of becoming passive has not. Their relative importance was established by Dung's original work,[1] which showed that 80.9% (80.5% in another of his studies) of a sample of 219 of his patients were at least mildly tender at T7. This point was followed in frequency by the other spinous processes: T5 (67.1%); T3 (41.1%); T6 (36.1%); T1 (19.2%); and T9 (17.8%). Thus, as the 112 acupoints throughout the body convert to the passive phase, these six midline points fall into that sequence. T7 is number 20 in that sequence; T5 is 39; T3 is 61; T6 is 64; T1 is 87; and T9 is 89.

Dung classified acupoints as primary, secondary, tertiary, and nonspecific. Generally, *primary acupoints* are those found to be passive in over 75% of individuals (actually, Dung studied individuals who presented to his clinic seeking acupuncture for painful conditions, so the percentages in the general population would be expected to be significantly lower). Using this standard, it can be seen that the spinous process of T7 is a primary point found to be passive in 80.9%. Similarly, *secondary acupoints* are those that Dung found to be passive in approximately 50 to 74% of his patient population — in this case T5. *Tertiary acupoints* are found to be passive in about 25 to 49% of the population, in this case T3 and T6. *Nonspecific acupoints* are found to be passive in less than 25% of individuals (T1 and T9).

Dung related these categories to an individual's lifetime accumulation of pain and the resulting progression of passive acupoints described in the previous chapter. The first systemic acupoints to become passive are the most important primary points: the Deep Radial-I, the Great Auricular, the Spinal Accessory-I, and so on as listed later in the next chapter. As an individual accumulates more pain, secondary acupoints begin to convert to the passive state, followed by the tertiary points, and finally by the nonspecific ones. The sequence of conversion is quite predictable for the primary points but becomes more variable for points further down the sequence; the secondary is more predictable than the tertiary and the tertiary more predictable than the nonspecific. This variation may be the

**TABLE 3.1**
**Pain Categories (Levels) and Quantification (Sensitivity)**

| Category (or "Level") | Pain Quantification (or "Sensitivity") |
|---|---|
| Primary | 1–3 |
| Secondary | 4–6 |
| Tertiary | 7–9 |
| Nonspecific | 10–12 |

result of regional exogenous factors or of variations in nerve characteristics (size, depth, etc.) among individuals.

The four *acupoint categories* (or *levels*) described previously are useful generalizations of the finer-grained 12-point pain sensitivity scale. These categories are related to pain quantification (sensitivity) as outlined in Table 3.1. The existence of these two scales can be more than a little confusing at first, so it is important to keep in mind the distinction between categories (or levels) and quantification (or sensitivity). It will be useful to keep in mind that sensitivity is indicated by the ordinal numbers 1 through 12, while categories are primary, secondary, etc. In clinical practice, the categories are generally more important than the exact quantification; the finer 12-point sensitivity scale is retained in this text because it may prove useful in future research. Sensitivity is often spoken of in conjunction with the term *degrees*, as in "Patient X has a pain sensitivity of five degrees, which makes her secondary."

As can be seen from this last example, categories (and levels) can apply to individuals as well as to points. It could be said that Patient X has most of the primary and some secondary points, but no tertiary or nonspecific ones, in the passive phase, so that finding makes her a secondary category individual. Dung thus divided individuals into the same four categories as he did points: primary, secondary, tertiary, and nonspecific. An individual is said to be *primary* if that person does not have any passive systemic acupoints beyond the primary level; *secondary* if he has passive primary and secondary acupoints but no tertiary ones; and *tertiary* if he has passive primary, secondary, and tertiary acupoints but no nonspecific ones. A person who has nonspecific systemic points in the passive phase is said to be *nonspecific*. Note that this discussion includes only systemic points; if a primary patient has a few nonspecific points around her recently sprained ankle, she is still in the primary category systemically. Dung found 27% of his pain patients to be primary; 35% to be secondary; 31% to be tertiary; and only 7% to be nonspecific. That these are not exact quartiles is not surprising, given the variability of the sequence, particularly as it applies to the less important acupoints.

The significance of a patient's level is profound. The level is highly predictive of a patient's likely response to acupuncture and to other attempts to manage pain. The primary patient is the patient who rarely has pain and, when he or she does, it is easily managed with over-the-counter analgesics. This patient will respond to almost any reasonable attempt to manage pain, including acupuncture, as long as no underlying structural abnormality (such as, in the knee, a torn meniscus) is perpetuating the pain. Paradoxically, this patient may tell the practitioner that he has a low pain threshold. If acupuncture is used to manage the pain, relatively few sessions (usually one to three) with relatively few needles inserted at each session are usually sufficient to obtain complete and lasting relief. Primary patients are often more sensitive to needles than are those at higher levels of pain sensitivity, and they are possibly more likely to fear needles. It may be that the psychological aspect of pain in these individuals reflects their relative lack of experience in handling pain; thus, pain is a newer experience for them and not easily ignored.

The secondary patient is harder to manage. This person may get temporary relief from over-the-counter medications, but the pain often recurs. Commonly, by the time this patient is seen in the acupuncture clinic, the pain has become chronic. He or she may require six acupuncture sessions utilizing more needles than would be required for a primary patient. Occasionally, these patients do not respond at all to acupuncture or require a greater number of sessions. Relief may be less than total, and repeated follow-up treatment (utilizing fewer sessions each time) may be required at 6- to 12-month intervals. These patients often say that they have high pain thresholds, often ignoring pain until it has progressed to the point that it is more difficult to manage. They may be "Type A" personalities subjected to sustained psychological stress (this is speculative, and an area deserving further study), or, as mentioned in the previous chapter, they may be women with a long history of dysmenorrhea.

The tertiary patient, especially the one with more than eight degrees of sensitivity, is extremely difficult to manage. This patient may often not find any pain relief except with narcotics. He or she is prone to develop many conditions spontaneously; examples are carpal tunnel syndrome and temporomandibular joint syndrome. The persistence of pain in these patients leads them frequently to devastating depression that may exacerbate the pain. These patients require many acupuncture sessions and have frequent relapses. One would think that they would abandon acupuncture as ineffective, but surprisingly they often seem to get some relief, and it is not unusual to have tertiary patients who have had hundreds of acupuncture treatments.

The nonspecific patient can rarely be helped. These patients often present for acupuncture having been diagnosed by another physician as having fibromyalgia. It has been our policy to explain the probability of failure to these prospective patients and to let them decide whether they want to try acupuncture. Occasionally, successes do occur, at least to some extent, after many treatment sessions; because many of these patients are desperate to try anything, we as practitioners are willing to give them the benefit of the doubt. Even if these patients do try, they may not come for enough treatments to get any benefit.

This broad range of individuals and their varied responses to acupuncture may help to explain why randomized controlled trials of acupuncture often produce equivocal results.

## 3.4 PAIN QUANTIFICATION USING REPRESENTATIVE ACUPOINTS (METHOD TWO)

As mentioned at the beginning of this chapter, the most direct and accurate method of determining the percentage of tender points on an individual's body is to palpate each of the 112 points and record the patient's response to each. This would require the practitioner to memorize the sequence of all 112 points or refer to a list, and to spend about an hour with each new patient to palpate and record all 112 points. Of course, this is impractical in a clinical setting. Fortunately, an easier method is available, but it requires the practitioner to memorize the sequence numbers of quite a few acupoints.

First of all, a few simple cautions should be considered before palpating acupoints. In a sensitive individual, the points can be quite tender, so the examiner should *be gentle.* Often patients will complain that "it didn't hurt until you pushed on it and made it hurt." Remember, only a force of about one kilogram of pressure is required, but if the examiner gets a positive tender reaction at a half kilogram of pressure, it is not necessary to apply more. How much force is required to produce a kilogram of pressure? The authors learned in the grocery store. While they were learning, they would place a thumb or forefinger in the middle of the basket of a produce scale and press until the scale registered two, then three, pounds, approximating a kilogram. In a very short time, applying the correct amount of pressure became second nature. If excessive pressure is used in assessing a patient, not only does the examiner arouse the patient's displeasure, but also the results of the assessment are skewed because any acupoint will be tender if enough pressure is applied to it.

Another caution is to verify the results obtained from one extremity by comparing that extremity to the opposite one. Generally, the 99 bilateral locations are the same sensitivity on either side of the body, but local factors such as a recent injury of one extremity may give artificially elevated results. Because generally an arm is examined first, it may be necessary to repeat the assessment on the other arm for comparison. If the results are inconsistent, one or both legs can be examined. Of course, many other

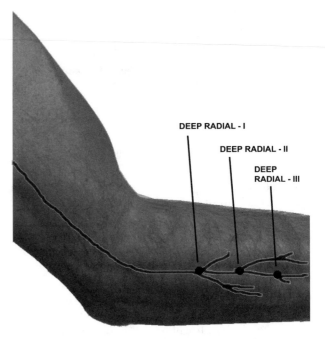

**FIGURE 3.2a** The Deep Radial-I (1), Deep Radial-II (29), and Deep Radial-III (79) acupoints fall along the deep radial nerve in the groove formed by the brachioradialis and extensor carpi radialis longus muscles.

points on the head and thorax may be examined as well, but if the assessment is confusing after examining all the extremities, it may be easier at this point to check the thoracic spinous processes as described in Method One.

To demonstrate how the system of representative acupoints works, consider the forearm (Figure 3.2a through Figure 3.2e). The forearm is quite accessible to the examiner and, when the weather is not too cool, usually exposed when the examiner first sees the patient. If it is not exposed, the examiner can ask the patient to push or roll up a sleeve, and several acupoints are immediately evident. The first acupoint to be examined in virtually all patients is the Deep Radial-I (1) point. The terminology indicates that, of several points along the deep radial nerve (deep radial points), this one is a primary point, as indicated by the "-I," and the number "1" in parentheses indicates that it is number one in the sequence of 112 acupoints. Usually, the sequence number is omitted in indicating the points, but is included here for convenience.

The Deep Radial-I (1) point is on the radial nerve, one of the large nerve trunks in the upper limb. The nerve supplies innervations to the extensor muscles of the arm. This point is found approximately 4 cm distal to the lateral epicondyle of the elbow in the groove formed by the brachioradialis and extensor carpi radialis longus muscles (Figure 3.2a). (As an exercise, the reader should find the Deep Radial-I (1) points on his or her forearms; they should be easy to find because they are most likely tender.)

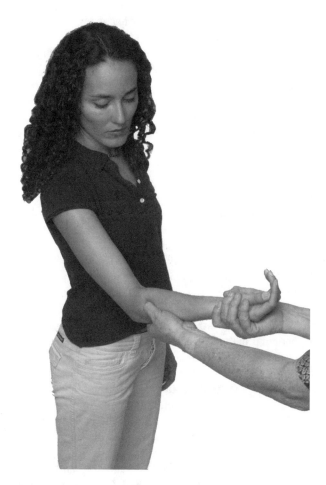

**FIGURE 3.2b** Palpating the Deep Radial-I (1) acupoint.

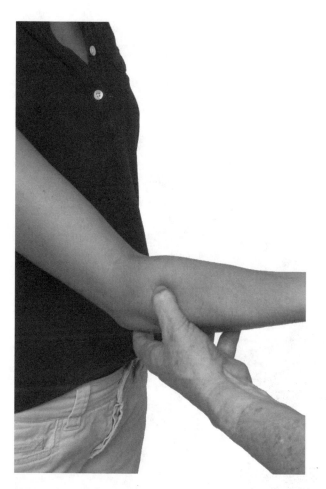

**FIGURE 3.2C** Close-up of Figure 3.2a.

The examiner should first have the patient totally relax the arm and palpate it as shown in Figure 3.2b and Figure 3.2c.

As the examiner palpates distally along this groove from the Deep Radial-I, another point will be found some 2 to 3 cm away: the Deep Radial-II (29). This point is easily located by palpating 2 to 3 cm distally from the Deep Radial-I along the groove formed by brachioradialis and extensor carpi radialis longus muscles (Figure 3.2a). Note that this point is the 29th in the sequence, making it a secondary point (There are 24 primary points, so this is the fifth in the sequence of the secondary points; the entire sequence will be enumerated in the following chapters). If a patient were to have all of his or her acupoints passive up to and including the Deep Radial-II point, but have no additional passive points, that patient would have a pain sensitivity of four on the 12-point scale. It can be seen from Table 3.2 that the Deep Radial-II point, with a sequence number of 29, falls within the secondary category with a pain quantification of four. Thus, if this point is tender, the patient is at least four degrees; if it is not, the patient is at most four degrees. If it is only slightly tender or significantly less tender than the Deep Radial-I, the patient is probably exactly four degrees. Simply by

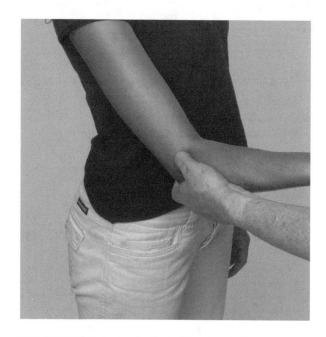

**FIGURE 3.2d** Palpating the Lateral Antebrachial Cutaneous (9) acupoint. Note that this is about 4 cm more proximal than the Deep Radial-I acupoint shown in Figure 3.2b and Figure 3.2c.

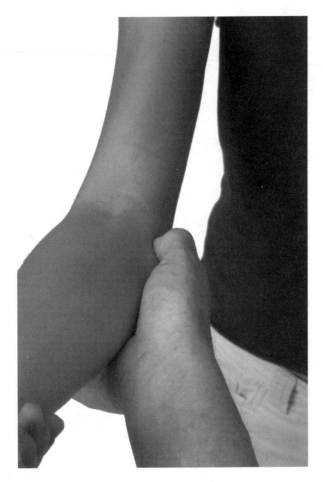

**FIGURE 3.2e** Palpating the Medial Antebrachial Cutaneous (25) acupoint.

**TABLE 3.2**
**Pain Categories and Quantification Related to Sequence Numbers of Passive Acupoints**

| Category | Pain Quantification (Degrees) | Points (Sequence Numbers) |
|---|---|---|
| Primary | 1 | 1–8 |
|  | 2 | 9–16 |
|  | 3 | 17–24 |
| Secondary | 4 | 25–33 |
|  | 5 | 34–42 |
|  | 6 | 43–52 |
| Tertiary | 7 | 53–61 |
|  | 8 | 62–70 |
|  | 9 | 71–79 |
| Nonspecific | 10–12 | 80–112 |

*Note:* The nonspecific category is too variable for exact sequence numbers to be meaningful.

palpating two points, the examiner has determined quite a bit of information.

From this table, it can be seen that a patient with only the Deep Radial-I (1) point in the passive phase would be in the primary category with a pain quantification of one. This patient might have total and permanent relief of pain after one to three acupuncture sessions as discussed earlier. A patient with each point passive up to and including the Deep Radial-II (29), but no more, would be in the secondary category with a pain quantification of four. This patient will most likely benefit from acupuncture after six to eight treatments, with relapses possible at 6- to 12-month intervals; because this patient is at the low end of the secondary category, this may be a somewhat pessimistic estimation of his or her prognosis.

The Deep Radial-III (79) is found another 2 to 3 cm down the deep radial nerve in the same groove (again, see Figure 3.2a). As can be seen from Table 3.2, this point is at the very end of the tertiary sequence. If this point is as tender as the other two deep radial points, then most likely the patient is in the nonspecific category and, if this finding is confirmed by examining other areas of the body, he or she is very unlikely to experience long-term benefit from acupuncture. In fact, the patient is unlikely to obtain relief from any other non-narcotic intervention to relieve pain.

Two other important acupoints in the forearm are the Lateral Antebrachial Cutaneous (9) and the Medial Antebrachial Cutaneous (25). (Because only one acupoint is along each of these nerves, the "-I" and "-II" suffixes are omitted.) The Medial Antebrachial Cutaneous (25) is important because it is the very first in the sequence of secondary points: a patient with this point tender is at least in the secondary category with a pain level of four. Similarly (refer to Table 3.2), the Lateral Antebrachial Cutaneous (9) point begins the second degree of pain quantification within the first category. Figure 3.2d and Figure 3.2e depict the palpation of these two acupoints.

In practice, the examiner will note a variation in a patient's response to palpation of different points, much as was described earlier in the discussion of the thoracic spinous processes, with some points more tender than others. For example, it would be typical to see that the Lateral Antebrachial Cutaneous (9) point is tenderer than the Medial Antebrachial Cutaneous (25). The significance of this finding is that it indicates that the tenderness of other secondary points further down the sequence will fall off rapidly; therefore, it would be acceptable to use this finding to estimate that the patient is not any higher than four degrees (five at the most). This could be confirmed by palpating a few more points, such as the Deep Radial-II (29). Also, it would be unlikely for the medial point to be tenderer because it is further down the sequence. An exception to this rule can be seen in this example: if the patient is suffering from medial epicondylitis ("backhand tennis elbow," "golfer's elbow"), this point may well be tenderer than the lateral one as a

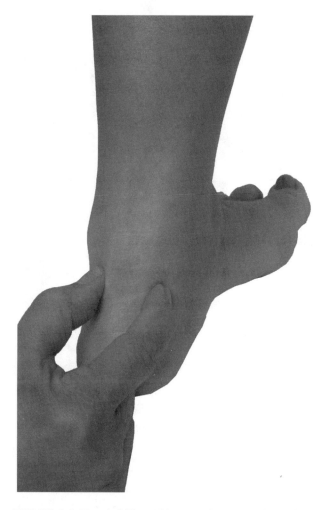

**FIGURE 3.3** The Achilles (54) acupoints used in patient assessment.

**TABLE 3.3**
**Rough Estimates of Pain Sensitivity Based on Palpation of Elbow and Forearm Alone[a]**

| DR-I (1)[b] | LAC (9)[c] | MAC (25)[d] | DR-II (29)[b] | DR-III (79)[b] | Sensitivity (Degree) |
|---|---|---|---|---|---|
| – | – | – | – | – | 0 |
| + | – | – | – | – | 1 |
| ++ | + | – | – | – | 2 |
| ++ | ++ | – or + | – | – | 3 |
| ++ | ++ | ++ | – or + | – | 4 |
| ++ | ++ | ++ | ++ | – | 5–8 |
| ++ | ++ | ++ | ++ | + | 9–10 |
| ++ | ++ | ++ | ++ | ++ | 10–12 |

[a] Slight tenderness is indicated by "+" and "++" indicates a greater degree of tenderness.
[b] DR = Deep Radial.
[c] LAC = Lateral Antebrachial Cutaneous.
[d] MAC = Medial Antebrachial Cutaneous.

local rather than a systemic response. The sequence being discussed is only relevant to systemic points.

The usefulness of this assessment technique cannot be underestimated. With no more than 1 or 2 minutes' worth of assessment, the patient has been placed in a category and, in the primary patient where differentiations between degrees are the most consistent and relevant, roughly within an exact degree. To summarize this point, Table 3.3 shows how precisely the sensitivity can be estimated using the elbow and forearm alone; the table indicates mild tenderness to standard palpation pressure as "+" and more marked tenderness to the same pressure as "++."

The main fault of this table based solely on the forearm is the lack of precision between the fifth and eighth degrees. Another point on another part of the body is required to complete the assessment, particularly in patients who seem to be somewhere in this range, i.e., they have a tender Deep Radial-II and a nontender Deep Radial-III. One might use one of the Achilles (54) points located on either side of the Achilles tendon (Figure 3.3); the "54" indicates that it is one of the first tertiary, seventh

degree points. Another useful point for this purpose is the Upper Biceps Brachii (55), a neuromuscular attachment of the musculocutaneous nerve located in the mass of the biceps muscle approximately one-third of the distance from the shoulder to the elbow along the anterior surface of the brachium (Figure 3.4).

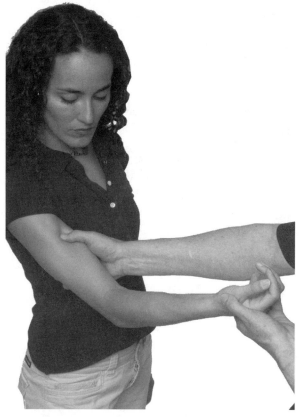

**FIGURE 3.4** The Upper Biceps Brachii (55) acupoint used in patient assessment.

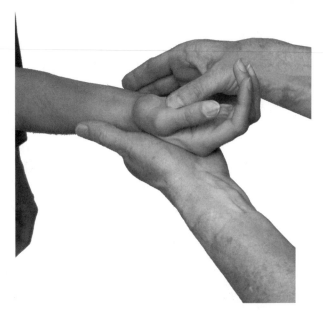

**FIGURE 3.5a** The Recurrent of Median (46) in the thenar eminence is palpated by the examiner's right thumb.

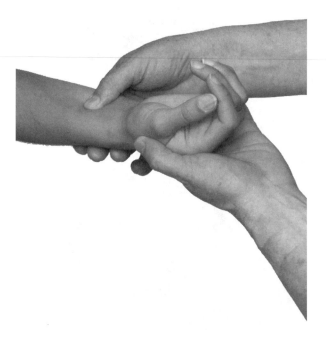

**FIGURE 3.5b** The Median (U) is palpated in the distal forearm.

Another means of estimation using only the forearm and hand involves checking the sensitivity of two additional points: one on the thenar eminence of the hand that is innervated by the recurrent of median nerve (Figure 3.5a) and the other, also innervated by the median nerve, in the midline of the anterior aspect of the forearm about 5 cm proximal to the proximal crease of the wrist (Figure 3.5b). If one of the two points is tender, the patient is probably secondary; if both are tender, the patient is more likely tertiary. (Because the recurrent of median nerve may enter the thenar eminence anywhere along the muscle mass, the examiner must "hunt around" for its associated acupoint.) Note that the described point on the volar aspect of the forearm is not numbered in the sequence; Dung failed to recognize the importance of that point when he conducted his earlier studies. It is most likely a secondary or tertiary point and will be indicated in this text as Median (U), the "U" representing "unknown."

Once the approximate anatomical location of an acupoint is understood, the point can easily be found by palpating in the general area until a tender spot is located; of course, if the point is in the latent phase, it cannot be found at all because it will not be tender to standard palpation pressure. Once again, it is advisable to check additional points to confirm one's initial impression; in a number of cases, individuals are very inconsistent and a few do not conform well to the sequence. In the following four chapters, all 112 acupoints are described and illustrated in order, with their gross and surface anatomical features described.

## REFERENCES

1. Dung, H.C. *Anatomical Acupuncture*. Antarctic Press, San Antonio, 1997.

# 4 The Primary Acupoints

## CONTENTS

## 4.1 INTRODUCTION

As their name implies, the primary points are the most important acupuncture points, so the acupuncture practitioner should memorize them. Their significance is that they are passive in most patients and, because the acupuncture treatment session usually consists of placing needles in passive acupoints, the primary points must be memorized as sites at which to insert needles. This general principle has two important limitations. First, the practitioner can only place needles in those points to which he has access; thus, it is typical to vary patient positioning from one session to the next so that over time more passive points are needled. The two most important positions are prone and supine, although the sitting and side positions are used frequently as well. Second, the number of needles that can or should be placed has a practical limit; it is unlikely that increasing the number of needles over 50 or so increases the efficacy of treatment, and patients have limits as to the numbers of needles they can tolerate in a single session.

Therefore, application of the general scheme has this significance: in a typical acupuncture session, needles are placed in local points relevant to the patient's pain, along with a realistic number of tender primary and secondary points that are accessible to the clinician. In the prone position, about 30 accessible primary points are accessible; adding passive secondary and local points relevant to the patient's source of pain, one can see that often 50 or more acupoints are candidates for needling. So, for example, in treating pain from a sprained ankle, local points around the ankle that have transitioned to the active or passive state would be needled, along with as many passive primary and secondary points as necessary, keeping the total number of needles within the patient's tolerance. If the patient has a pain sensitivity of zero (signifying that he has no primary or secondary points in the passive phase), it is not necessary to needle *any* primary or secondary points, just those around the ankle. From this dis-

cussion, it can be seen that at least some primary points are needled in nearly every session for most patients.

In the list that follows, the percentages of patients from Dung's earlier work[1] found to have these points in the passive phase are indicated in parentheses after the names of the points. More information will be given about these points in subsequent chapters describing acupuncture in specific anatomic regions of the body. The main purpose of this chapter and the three that follow is to assist the reader in anatomically locating the points. It should be remembered that these points can be easily located in most individuals by palpating for tenderness. The reader is advised to combine palpation with the descriptions that follow to locate these important acupoints, and to consult a reliable anatomical atlas (while exercising caution because most atlases do not portray peripheral — especially cutaneous — nerves with much precision).

Figures throughout this text use a star symbol to depict primary points.

## 4.2 PRIMARY ACUPOINTS

The primary acupoints are presented in sequence of their becoming passive (Figure 4.1a and Figure 4.1b):

1. Deep Radial-I (99.5% of pain patients have this point in the passive phase). The point is derived from the postaxial (or posterior) division of the brachial plexus, which derives from the ventral primary rami of C5, C6, C7, C8, and T1. Because of the rotation of the forearm during embryologic development, the flexor compartment moves from an anterior position to the ulnar or medial side while the extensor compartment moves to the radial or lateral side. The deep radial nerve enters the lateral (extensor) compartment of the forearm to supply the extensor muscles of the wrist and fingers. The

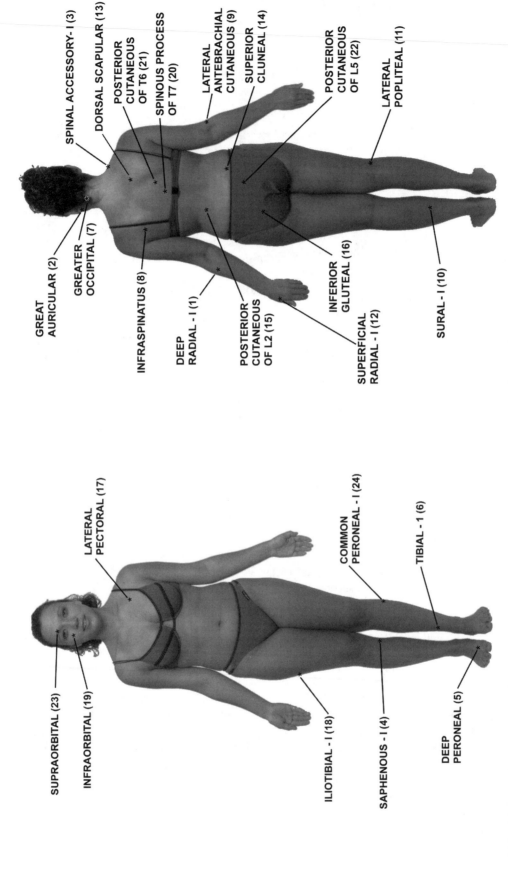

**FIGURE 4.1b** Primary acupoints indicated by sequence numbers: posterior aspect.

**FIGURE 4.1a** Primary acupoints indicated by sequence numbers: anterior aspect

nerve branches and sends innervations to the individual muscles of the extensor compartment at the intermuscular septum separating the brachioradialis from the other muscles of the compartment — specifically, the extensor carpi radialis longus. In a muscular person, the septum can be distinguished as a groove running longitudinally along the muscle mass of the lateral side of the forearm. (This was pictured in the previous chapter, particularly in Figure 3.2a.) The nerve first branches approximately 4 cm distal to the lateral epicondyle, creating the Deep Radial-I acupoint. Other acupoints appear distally every 2 to 3 cm along this nerve; these are more minor points, reflecting the decreasing caliber of the nerve, that will be described in the next two chapters. See Figure 4.1b and Figure 4.4b.

2. Great Auricular (99.1%). This acupoint is formed by the great auricular nerve, which is one of four named cutaneous branches of the cervical nerve plexus arising from the ventral primary rami of C1, C2, C3, and C4. It emerges at the midpoint of the posterior border of the sternocleidomastoid muscle along with the other three cutaneous branches of the cervical plexus, and then turns upward on the sternocleidomastoid muscle obliquely in a course toward the auricle (earlobe) and the angle of the mandible. The nerve bundle then pierces the deep investing fascia and forms this acupoint, which is detected by placing a finger just behind the lowest point of the earlobe. See Figure 4.1b, Figure 4.2a, Figure 4.2b, and Figure 4.4b.

3. Spinal Accessory-I (98.2%). This is the 11th cranial nerve that innervates two muscles, the trapezius and the sternocleidomastoid. Two potential acupoints are formed by the neuromuscular attachments to these two muscles, but in practice only the attachment to the trapezius is significant. This point is located over the medial portion of the muscle mass on the top of the shoulder. Often a hard nodule can be palpated at this point. Additional points may form around this point and more laterally along the superior aspect of the shoulder as will be seen later. When this point is needled, particularly in thin individuals, care should be used to keep from entering the pleural cavity and creating a pneumothorax; in an individual of normal muscle mass, however, this is extremely unlikely. See Figure 4.1b, Figure 4.2a, Figure 4.2b, Figure 4.3b, and Figure 4.4b.

4. Saphenous-I (97.7%). The femoral nerve, the largest branch of the lumbar plexus (from the anterior primary rami of L2 through L4),

becomes the saphenous nerve after it emerges inferomedially from underneath the sartorius muscle and pierces the deep fascia at the medial side of the knee. It becomes very superficial under the medial condyle of the tibia where it becomes a cutaneous nerve innervating the medial surface of the leg as far as the medial malleolus. Five acupoints are formed by the nerve on the medial aspect of the leg: one posterior and four others along the posterior margin of the tibia following the course of the nerve. The posterior point is situated somewhat behind the condyle, while the four others are more anterior and distal to the condyle. The most superior of the four distal points is the Saphenous-I, with the others falling more distally and somewhat anteriorly along the posterior border of the tibia. The Saphenous-I is easily palpated in most persons as a tender point some 2 cm distal to the medial condyle and 2 cm posterior to the medial aspect of the tibia. See Figure 4.1a and Figure 4.5a.

5. Deep Peroneal (97.3%). The deep peroneal nerve is a cutaneous nerve arising from the common peroneal, which arises from the lateral branch of the sciatic nerve (derived from the sacral nerve plexus). The Deep Peroneal acupoint is found approximately 1 to 2 cm proximal to the web between the great and second toes and between those toes' extensor tendons. See Figure 4.1a and Figure 4.5a.

6. Tibial-I (96.8%). The tibial nerve, a branch of the sciatic nerve giving off cutaneous and muscular branches, comes close to the skin about 6 to 7 cm above the medial malleolus and posterior to the tibia; there it divides into two plantar nerves and forms an important acupoint. See Figure 4.1a and Figure 4.5a.

7. Greater Occipital (96.4%). This nerve arises from the posterior primary ramus of C2. It is a sensory nerve that becomes subcutaneous approximately 2 or 3 cm lateral to the external occipital protuberance and slightly below it. See Figure 4.1b and Figure 4.2b.

8. Infraspinatus (95.9%). This is one of two acupoints of the suprascapular nerve; the other is the supraspinatus (49). This nerve arises from the postaxial division of the brachial plexus. The acupoint is found at the nerve's neuromuscular attachment to the infraspinatus muscle, a broad muscle with a thin mass. The nerve enters the muscle near the center of the infraspinatus fossa to establish the neuromuscular attachment and acupoint. See Figure 4.1b, Figure 4.2b, Figure 4.3b, and Figure 4.4b. (Dung's original work named this point the "Suprascapular-I.")[1]

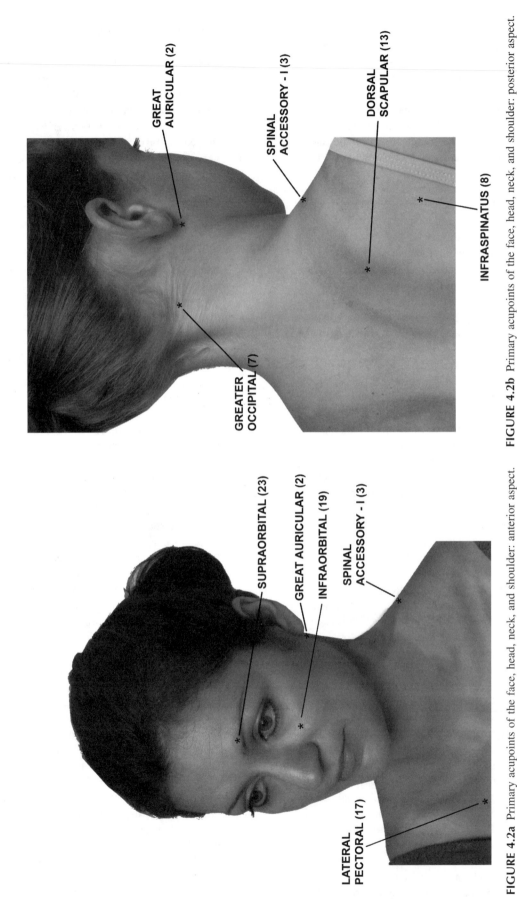

GREAT
AURICULAR (2)

SPINAL
ACCESSORY - I (3)

DORSAL
SCAPULAR (13)

INFRASPINATUS (8)

GREATER
OCCIPITAL (7)

**FIGURE 4.2b** Primary acupoints of the face, head, neck, and shoulder: posterior aspect.

SUPRAORBITAL (23)

GREAT AURICULAR (2)

INFRAORBITAL (19)

SPINAL
ACCESSORY - I (3)

LATERAL
PECTORAL (17)

**FIGURE 4.2a** Primary acupoints of the face, head, neck, and shoulder: anterior aspect.

9. Lateral Antebrachial Cutaneous (95.5%). This is a branch of the musculocutaneous nerve that pierces the deep fascia at the lateral edge of the cubital fossa. The point is most easily found by having the patient flex the elbow maximally and then locating the point at the lateral end of the elbow crease. See Figure 4.1b and Figure 4.4b.

10. Sural-I (94.6%). The sural nerve is formed by union of the lateral sural branch of the common peroneal nerve and the medial sural branch of the tibial nerve. It supplies innervation to the skin of the lateral and posterior portions of the distal one third of the leg. Its major acupoint is formed at the distal margin of the mass of the two heads of the gastrocnemius muscle in the midline of the posterior surface of the leg. When placing a needle in this point, it is helpful to stay in line with the Achilles tendon at the foot. See Figure 4.1b and Figure 4.5b.

11. Lateral Popliteal (93.7%). The Lateral and Medial Popliteal points are exceptional. Located in the popliteal fossa, one or the other of them (mostly the lateral) is used every time a patient is needled in the prone position. The Lateral Popliteal acupoint is located just medial to the tendon of the short head of the biceps femoris; no important cutaneous nerve is associated with it. A branch of the posterior femoral cutaneous nerve is nearby but not exactly at the location of the acupoint. The common peroneal nerve is deep to the point and may have its division into the superficial and deep peroneal branches at this site. See Figure 4.1b and Figure 4.5b.

Dung in his earlier work does not list the Medial Popliteal point in the sequence, but in practice uses the point interchangeably with the Lateral Popliteal. The medial point is just lateral to the tendons of the semitendinosus and semimembranosus muscles in the popliteal fossa and, curiously, is more tender in younger persons (e.g., less than 20 years old) than the lateral one; as a person ages, the lateral point becomes more likely to become tender and the medial one less so. When Dung needles a patient in the prone position then, he needles the medial point in younger patients and the lateral one in older ones.

12. Superficial Radial-I (91.9%). The superficial radial nerve emerges from under the brachioradialis muscle at the distal radius. Acupoints can appear from the point of emergence throughout the length of the nerve, often in response to a neuropathy caused by an injury to the nerve such as a blow to the radius near the wrist. The nerve does not branch until it reaches the anatomic snuffbox, where a minor acupoint can form, and the web between the thumb and index finger. The most important acupoint for the superficial radial nerve is exactly in the middle of the web. See Figure 4.1b and Figure 4.4b.

13. Dorsal Scapular (91.0%). This nerve is derived from the postaxial division of the brachial plexus to innervate three muscles: the levator scapulae; the rhomboid major; and the rhomboid minor. It descends from the cervical region down to the medial border of the scapula, where it enters the muscle mass to form a neuromuscular attachment and acupoint approximately 1 cm superior to the base of the spine of the scapula. The point is actually slightly beneath the margin of the scapula and should be needled with the point of the needle directed at a slight lateral angle to slide beneath the bone, taking care to avoid inserting the needle so deeply as to create a pneumothorax. See Figure 4.1b, Figure 4.2b, Figure 4.3b, and Figure 4.4b.

14. Superior Cluneal (89.6%). Derived from the dorsal primary rami of the first three lumbar spinal nerves, this cutaneous nerve pierces the thoracolumbar fascia at the highest point of the iliac crest posteriorly. The acupoint is deep, especially in obese individuals, and is best palpated by pressing over the top of the crest to penetrate deeply and inferiorly beneath the margin of the bone; it should be needled with long needles angled inferiorly over the top of the crest to reach the point. This point is almost always tender in patients complaining of low back pain. See Figure 4.1b, Figure 4.3b, and Figure 4.4b.

15. Posterior Cutaneous of L2 (88.7%). This point is located along the posterior waistline approximately 6 cm lateral to the midline, where the lateral branch of L2 penetrates the thoracolumbar fascia lateral to the erector spinae muscles. This important point is used to treat low back pain. See Figure 4.1b, Figure 4.3b, and Figure 4.4b.

16. Inferior Gluteal (88.2%). The inferior gluteal nerve arises from the posterior branches of the anterior primary rami of the fifth lumbar spinal nerve and the first two sacral spinal nerves. It leaves the pelvis through the greater sciatic foramen below the piriformis and enters the gluteus maximus muscle. The muscle is large and thick and the nerve is deep within it, yielding only one acupoint. This Inferior Gluteal point is located right in the center of the gluteal region, where the nerve enters the gluteus maximus muscle to form a neuromuscular attachment.

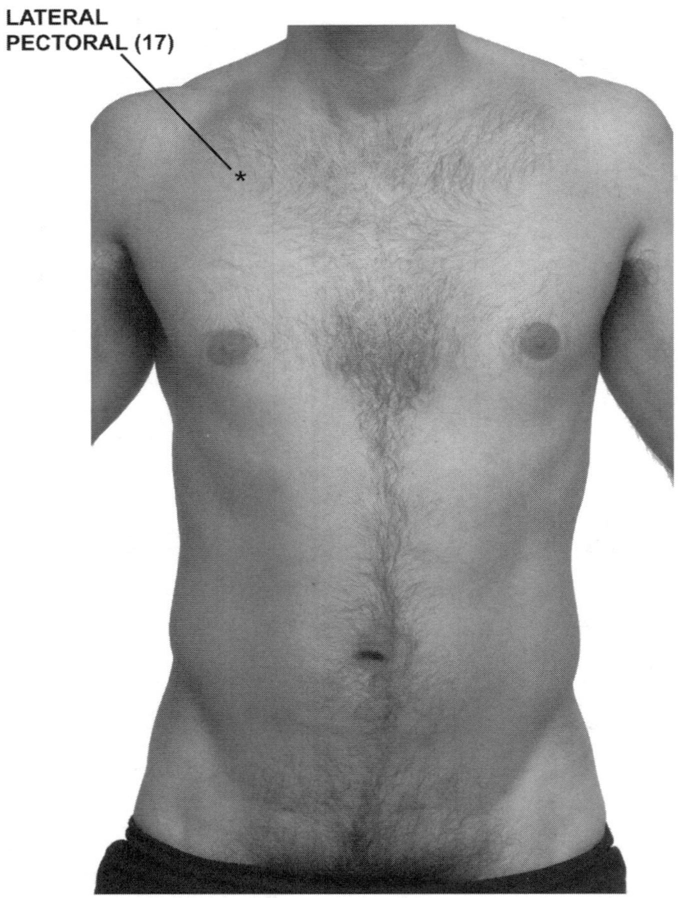

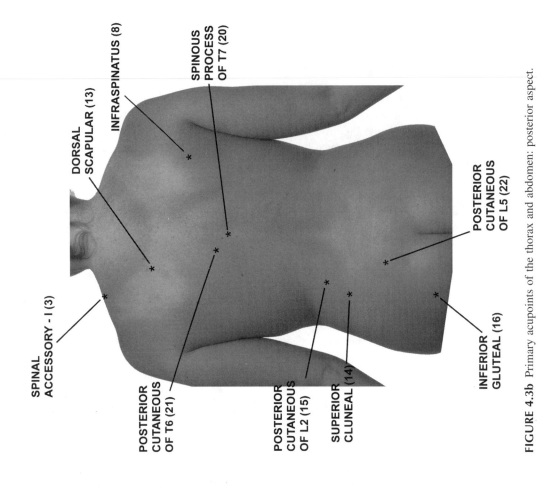

SPINAL
ACCESSORY - I (3)

DORSAL
SCAPULAR (13)

INFRASPINATUS (8)

SPINOUS
PROCESS
OF T7 (20)

POSTERIOR
CUTANEOUS
OF T6 (21)

POSTERIOR
CUTANEOUS
OF L2 (15)

SUPERIOR
CLUNEAL (14)

POSTERIOR
CUTANEOUS
OF L5 (22)

INFERIOR
GLUTEAL (16)

**FIGURE 4.3b** Primary acupoints of the thorax and abdomen: posterior aspect.

LATERAL
PECTORAL (17)

**FIGURE 4.3a** Primary acupoints of the thorax and abdomen: anterior aspect.

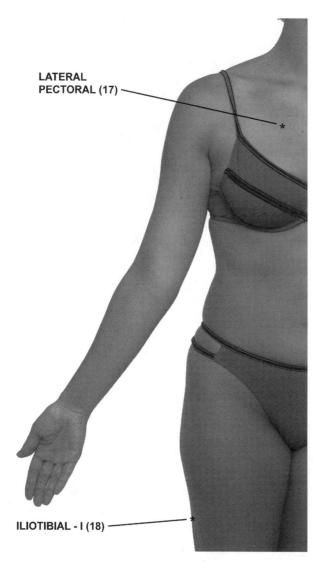

FIGURE 4.4a Primary acupoints of the upper extremity: anterior aspect.

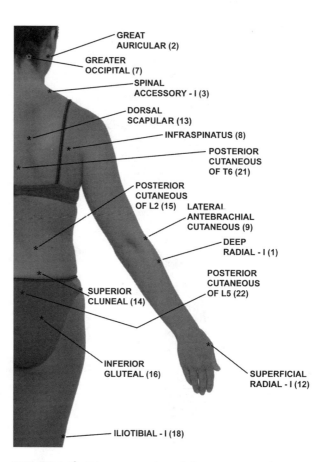

FIGURE 4.4b Primary acupoints of the upper extremity: posterior aspect.

Pain in this acupoint often is erroneously attributed to the piriformis muscle (so-called piriformis syndrome).[2] Although the point may become a tender local point in response to regional injury, it is unlikely that pain is created by direct pressure on the nerve by surrounding structures, as is commonly proposed. See Figure 4.1b, Figure 4.3b, Figure 4.4b, and Figure 4.5b.

17. Lateral Pectoral (86.9%). The lateral pectoral nerve is derived from the anterior division of the ventral primary rami of the spinal nerves of the brachial plexus. The acupoint is the neuromuscular attachment of the nerve to the pectoralis major muscle. It is found 4 cm inferior to the middle of the clavicle or slightly more medially. When inserting needles into the chest wall, care should be taken not to penetrate so deeply

as to puncture the pleura and create a pneumothorax. See Figure 4.1a, Figure 4.2a, Figure 4.3a, and Figure 4.4a.

18. Iliotibial-I (83.7%). These cutaneous nerves, which come directly from the sciatic nerve deep in the thigh, are not described in anatomy texts, but have been frequently observed by author Dung, as described in his earlier work on acupuncture.[1] He describes most cadavers as having four of these nerves penetrating the iliotibial tract along the lateral thigh where their associated acupoints are found. Iliotibial-I (18) is found approximately in the middle of the length of the tract. These acupoints are useful in treating meralgia paraesthetica (pain occurring on the lateral surface of the thigh). Dung in his earlier work cast doubt on the commonly accepted role of the lateral femoral cutaneous nerve in producing meralgia paraesthetica. See Figure 4.1a, Figure 4.4a, Figure 4.4b, Figure 4.5a, and Figure 4.5b.

19. Infraorbital (83.3%). The infraorbital nerve emerges through the infraorbital foramen of the maxilla, the largest foramen of the face, to become cutaneous and form an acupoint just

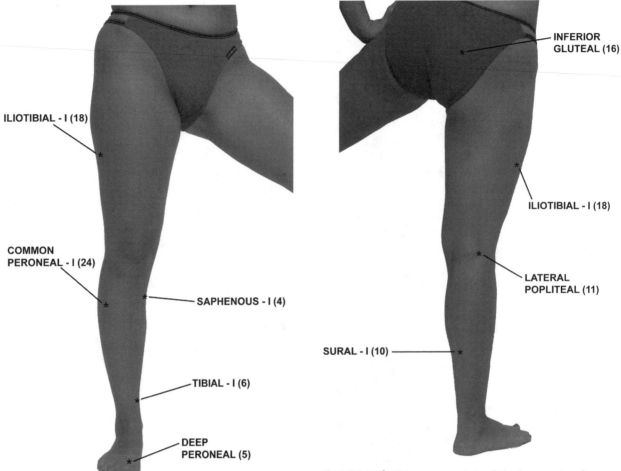

**FIGURE 4.5a** Primary acupoints of the lower extremity: anterior aspect.

**FIGURE 4.5b** Primary acupoints of the lower extremity: posterior aspect.

below the inferior rim of the orbital fossa. This is the most important acupoint of the face and is essential in managing headache. It is located superficial to the foramen approximately 2 cm below the inferior eyelid and 2 cm lateral to the lateral margin of the nose. When needling acupoints in the face, it is neither necessary nor desirable to insert needles into the foramina — simply piercing the skin superficially is adequate. The foramen is crowded and wedging a needle into it could damage the nerve or its accompanying blood vessels. See Figure 4.1a and Figure 4.2a.

20. Spinous Process of T7 (80.5%). This point was described in the previous chapter's discussion of pain quantification using thoracic spinous processes (method one). It is formed by the ligamentum nuchae, an expansion of the supraspinous ligament that joins the tips of the spinous processes. T7 is located in the midpoint

of a line joining the inferior angles of the scapulae. See Figure 4.1b and Figure 4.3b.

21. Posterior Cutaneous of T6 (77.8%). The posterior primary rami of T6 form two terminal cutaneous nerves, which for acupuncture purposes can be treated as one point, 2 to 3 cm lateral to the T6 spinous process. This point is seldom palpated clinically but is often needled therapeutically. When this point is needled, care should be taken, especially in thin individuals, to avoid creating a pneumothorax. See Figure 4.1b, Figure 4.3b, and Figure 4.4b.

22. Posterior Cutaneous of L5 (76.0%). Although this nerve is called "cutaneous" to maintain consistency with the names of posterior primary rami of nerves higher in the spine, L4 and L5 are thought to have no cutaneous branches. This would be more properly called the muscular branch of the posterior primary ramus of L5. The point is formed at the neuromuscular attachment with the erector spinae muscles 4 to

5 cm lateral to the L5 spinous process. See Figure 4.1b, Figure 4.3b, and Figure 4.4b.

23. Supraorbital (75.6%). The Supraorbital point is formed at the site where the supraorbital nerve emerges through the supraorbital foramen. The foramen is the second largest of those of the face and the supraorbital nerve is the second largest in nerve mass in the face. Not surprisingly, the acupoint at the emergence of the nerve through the foramen is the second facial acupoint to become tender in the progression of pain. To locate this point, visualize the eyebrow as divided into thirds; this point is located between the medial and middle thirds on the superior margin of the eyebrow. The supraorbital artery and vein accompany the nerve at this point. The autonomic fibers mixed with the supraorbital nerve arise from the superior cervical ganglion of the sympathetic nervous system. As with the Infraorbital (19) point, it is neither necessary nor desirable to insert needles into the foramina — simply piercing the skin superficially is adequate. See Figure 4.1a and Figure 4.2a.

24. Common Peroneal-I (74.7%). The common peroneal nerve (called "fibular" in some texts) arises from the lateral branch of the sciatic nerve. At the superior angle of the popliteal fossa, the nerve follows the medial border of the biceps femoris muscle and its tendon along the superolateral boundary of the fossa, where it leaves the fossa by passing superficially to the lateral head of the gastrocnemius muscle. It then passes over the back of the head of the fibula before winding around the lateral surface of the neck of the bone. The nerve finally runs beneath the upper fibers of the peroneus longus muscle to enter the lateral compartment of the leg. At the head of the fibula and posterolateral to its neck, the nerve can be palpated by rolling it against the bone. It then bifurcates into the superficial and deep peroneal nerves in the proximal region of the lateral compartment where it forms an important point, the Common Peroneal-I (24). The point is best located by palpating the head of the fibula and then moving 2 or 3 cm inferomedially. Additional, less important points are located along the distal course of the nerve, as will be seen in the following chapters. See Figure 4.1a and Figure 4.5a.

## REFERENCES

1. Dung, H.C. *Anatomical Acupuncture.* Antarctic Press, San Antonio, 1997.
2. Fitzgerald, R.H., Kaufer, H., Malkani, A.L., et al. *Orthopaedics,* Mosby, St. Louis, 2002: 874.

# 5 The Secondary Acupoints

## CONTENTS

## 5.1 INTRODUCTION

Secondary acupoints are also important, but not as important as the primary points. They are more frequently needled in an area of regional pain. For example, in a patient with carpal tunnel syndrome, it would be appropriate to needle the recurrent of median (46) point *in both extremities* — the affected and the unaffected. (The authors believe there is a tendency for some painful conditions without structural derangement to manifest bilaterally as they progress, making it prudent to needle the unaffected side prophylactically.)

The secondary acupoints in this chapter are arranged like those in the previous one, with the sequence numbers followed by the name of the point and, in parentheses, the percentage of Dung's patients in his previously published series having the point in the passive phase. Figures throughout this text use a square symbol to depict secondary points (the star symbol is used to designate primary points).

## 5.2 SECONDARY ACUPOINTS

The secondary acupoints are presented in the sequence of their becoming passive (Figure 5.1a and Figure 5.1b):

25. Medial Antebrachial Cutaneous (74.6%). This nerve is located on the medial aspect of the elbow, slightly anterior to the medial epicondyle on the medial end of the cubital fossa; it derives from the medial cord of the brachial plexus (C8 and T1) and is accompanied by the basilic vein. See Figure 5.1a and Figure 5.4a, and also Figure 3.2e in the chapter on pain quantification.

26. Tibial-II (74.6%). This is 2 to 3 cm distal to the Tibial-I (6). See Figure 5.1a and Figure 5.5a, and the discussion of the Tibial-I (6) acupoint in the previous chapter.

27. Temporomandibular (74.6%). This is the lowest of a linear triad of points just anterior to the ear (the other two are called the Auriculotemporal (U) and the Anterior Auricular (U) points), progressing caudally from the temporomandibular point. The Temporomandibular, innervated by the mandibular branch of the trigeminal nerve (the fifth cranial nerve), is over the temporomandibular joint (TMJ). The three points of the triad are secondary, tertiary, and nonspecific as they progress superiorly. The Auriculotemporal and Anterior Auricular points were not included in Dung's original research establishing the sequence of 112 acupoints, so they will not be found in subsequent chapters as numbered points. They are nonetheless important and will be discussed later in the text in conjunction with conditions of the face and head. See Figure 5.1a, Figure 5.2a, and Figure 5.2b for the location of the Temporomandibular point. The Auriculotemporal point is approximately 2 cm above the Temporomandibular point, and the Anterior Auricular is 2 cm above the Auriculotemporal.

28. Cervical Plexus (74.2%). Derived from the interconnecting branches of the ventral primary rami of the first four cervical spinal nerves, this point is formed where the four cutaneous branches of the cervical plexus emerge from beneath the muscle layer at the midpoint of the posterior border of the sternocleidomastoid muscle. It is easily found by placing a thumb on the sternoclavicular joint and the index finger on the mastoid process; the acupoint is at the midpoint between these two locations. It is on the anterior margin of the posterior triangle and is fairly deep, but represents a fairly large congregation of fibers, making it an important acupoint. See Figure 5.1a, Figure 5.2a, and Figure 5.2b.

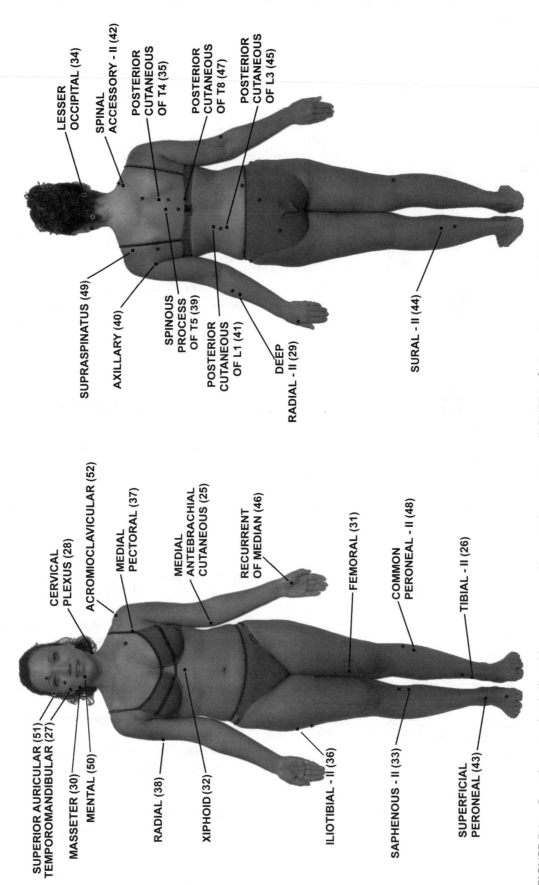

LESSER OCCIPITAL (34)
SPINAL ACCESSORY - II (42)
POSTERIOR CUTANEOUS OF T4 (35)
POSTERIOR CUTANEOUS OF T8 (47)
POSTERIOR CUTANEOUS OF L3 (45)

SUPRASPINATUS (49)
AXILLARY (40)
SPINOUS PROCESS OF T5 (39)
POSTERIOR CUTANEOUS OF L1 (41)
DEEP RADIAL - II (29)
SURAL - II (44)

**FIGURE 5.1b**  Secondary acupoints indicated by sequence numbers: posterior aspect.

CERVICAL PLEXUS (28)
ACROMIOCLAVICULAR (52)
MEDIAL PECTORAL (37)
MEDIAL ANTEBRACHIAL CUTANEOUS (25)
RECURRENT OF MEDIAN (46)
FEMORAL (31)
COMMON PERONEAL - II (48)
TIBIAL - II (26)

SUPERIOR AURICULAR (51)
TEMPOROMANDIBULAR (27)
MASSETER (30)
MENTAL (50)
RADIAL (38)
XIPHOID (32)
ILIOTIBIAL - II (36)
SAPHENOUS - II (33)
SUPERFICIAL PERONEAL (43)

**FIGURE 5.1a**  Secondary acupoints indicated by sequence numbers: anterior aspect.

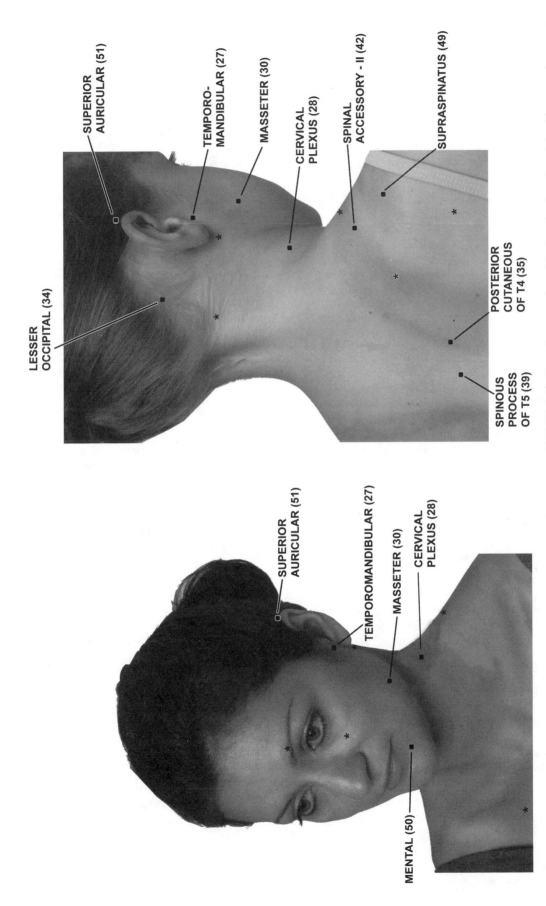

**FIGURE 5.2b** Secondary acupoints of the face, head, neck, and shoulder: posterior aspect.

**FIGURE 5.2a** Secondary acupoints of the face, head, neck, and shoulder: anterior aspect.

29. Deep Radial-II (74.2%). This is 2 to 3 cm distal to the Deep Radial-I (1). See Figure 5.1b and Figure 5.4b, Figure 3.2a in the chapter on pain quantification, and the discussion of the Deep Radial-I (1) point in the previous chapter.

30. Masseter (73.6%). This acupoint from the mandibular branch of the trigeminal nerve (the fifth cranial nerve) is about 2 cm anterior to and cephalad from the mandibular angle and is the neuromuscular attachment of the masseter muscle. The nerve to this muscle passes over the mandibular notch to enter the inner surface of the muscle, where its small and deep fibers form the point. The masseter nerve is considered a muscular one, but it contains efferent and afferent fibers that give it a more complex composition than a pure muscular nerve. See Figure 5.1a, Figure 5.2a, and Figure 5.2b.

31. Femoral (72.9%). This cutaneous branch of the femoral nerve forms an acupoint about 7 cm proximal to the medial condyle of the tibia. See Figure 5.1a and Figure 5.5a.

32. Xiphoid (72.4%). This is innervated by the anterior cutaneous nerves of T5, which circle the trunk from the spine and terminate just lateral to the anterior midline over the xiphoid process of the sternum. See Figure 5.1a and Figure 5.3a.

33. Saphenous-II (70.6%). This is approximately 2 to 3 cm distal to the Saphenous-I (4). See Figure 5.1a, Figure 5.5a, and the discussion of Saphenous-I (4) in the previous chapter.

34. Lesser Occipital (68.8%). Innervated by the lesser occipital nerve coursing along the posterior border of the sternocleidomastoid muscle from the cervical plexus, this point is located behind the mastoid process at the superior posterior margin of the sternocleidomastoid muscle. See Figure 5.1b, Figure 5.2b, and Figure 5.4b.

35. Posterior Cutaneous of T4 (67.0%). This is located 2 to 3 cm lateral to the T4 spinous process. There is a pneumothorax risk in needling this point too deeply. See Figure 5.1b, Figure 5.2b, Figure 5.3b, Figure 5.4b, and the discussion of the Posterior Cutaneous of T6 (21) acupoint in the previous chapter.

36. Iliotibial-II (66.5%). This is approximately 5 to 6 cm proximal to the Iliotibial-I (18) along the iliotibial tract. See Figure 5.1a, Figure 5.4a, Figure 5.4b, Figure 5.5a, Figure 5.5b, and the discussion of Iliotibial-I (18) in the previous chapter.

37. Medial Pectoral (66.1%). This is approximately 4 cm inferolateral to the Lateral Pectoral (17). It is formed by the neuromuscular attachment of the medial pectoral nerve to the pectoralis major muscle. Because the nerve is smaller but otherwise similar to that of the Lateral Pectoral (17), the point becomes tender later in the sequence than the Lateral Pectoral. This point is a pneumothorax risk if needled too deeply. See Figure 5.1a, Figure 5.3a, and Figure 5.4a.

38. Radial (64.7%). This is one of the large nerve trunks in the upper limb supplying the extensor muscles of the arm. After leaving the axillary region, the radial nerve runs downward, backward, and laterally between the long and medial heads of the triceps to enter the radial groove of the humerus. The trunk of the radial nerve can be palpated at the location where it lies in the groove immediately below the insertion of the deltoid muscle on the lateral surface of the brachium (upper arm). At this, the location of the Radial (38) acupoint, the radial nerve gives off the posterior antebrachial cutaneous nerve supplying the skin of the posterior surface of the forearm. This is not a very important point because of its depth. Note that it is not the same as the Deep Radial points. See Figure 5.1a and Figure 5.4b.

39. Spinous Process of T5 (64.3%; 67.1% in another series described by Dung*). This is the T5 equivalent of the Spinous Process of T7 (20) point, discussed in the previous two chapters. See Figure 5.1b, Figure 5.2b, and Figure 5.3b.

40. Axillary (62.4%). The axillary nerve passes through the quadrangular space to reach the back of the shoulder joint. The nerve winds around the surgical neck of the humerus and innervates the teres minor and deltoid muscles. The axillary nerve forms an acupoint at the peak of the posterior axillary fold. Branches of the axillary nerve entering the teres minor and the deltoid can also contribute neuromuscular attachments to form acupoints. See Figure 5.1b, Figure 5.3b, and Figure 5.4b.

41. Posterior Cutaneous of L1 (62.4%). This is the L1 equivalent of the Posterior Cutaneous of L2 (15) acupoint. See Figure 5.1b, Figure 5.3b, Figure 5.4b, and the discussion of the Posterior Cutaneous of L2 (15) acupoint in the previous chapter

42. Spinal Accessory-II (61.1%). This point is indicated in Figure 5.1b, Figure 5.2b, Figure

---

* This second series was the one in which Dung derived the quantification method using thoracic spinous processes, described as method one in Chapter 3. In his earlier text cited elsewhere, Dung described two major series of patients: one was used to develop the sequence of 112 (actually 110) acupoints and the other was used to develop the thoracic spinous process method.

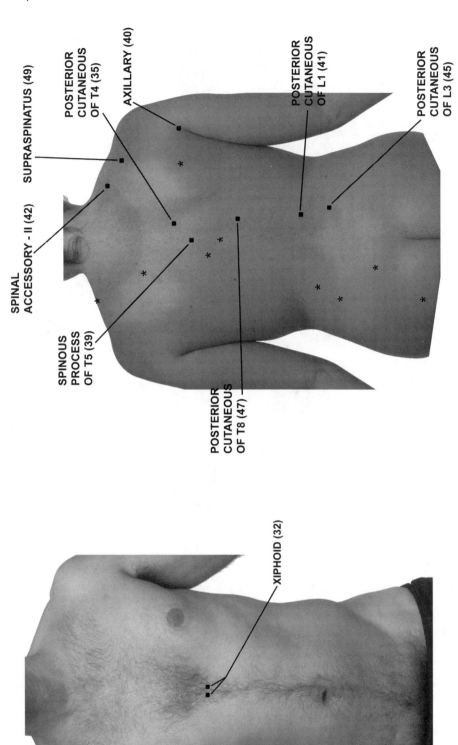

**SUPRASPINATUS (49)**

**POSTERIOR CUTANEOUS OF T4 (35)**

**AXILLARY (40)**

**POSTERIOR CUTANEOUS OF L1 (41)**

**POSTERIOR CUTANEOUS OF L3 (45)**

**SPINAL ACCESSORY - II (42)**

**SPINOUS PROCESS OF T5 (39)**

**POSTERIOR CUTANEOUS OF T8 (47)**

**FIGURE 5.3b** Secondary acupoints of the thorax and abdomen: posterior aspect.

**XIPHOID (32)**

**MEDIAL PECTORAL (37)**

**FIGURE 5.3a** Secondary acupoints of the thorax and abdomen: anterior aspect.

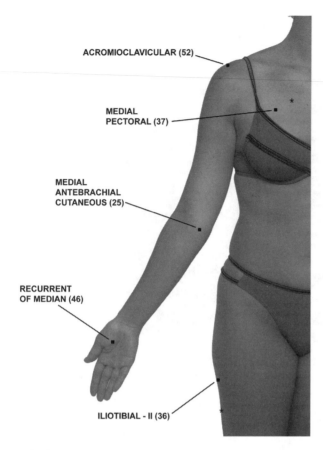

**FIGURE 5.4a** Secondary acupoints of the upper extremity: anterior aspect.

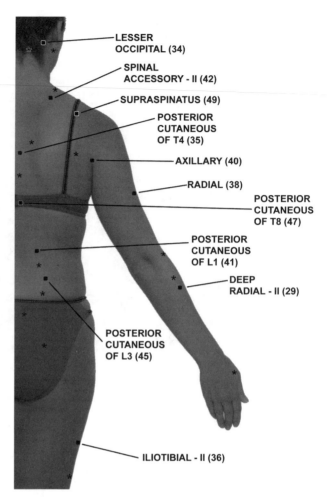

**FIGURE 5.4b** Secondary acupoints of the upper extremity: posterior aspect.

5.3b, and Figure 5.4b as being about 2 cm inferior to the Spinal Accessory-I (3). In reality, a secondary point of the spinal accessory nerve can occur anywhere in the area of Spinal Accessory-I within a radius of 2 or 3 cm. The most common locations for a secondary point to appear are inferior or lateral. To find this point in an individual, first find the Spinal Accessory-I and then palpate around it within the specified radius to see if another point can be found. This point poses a pneumothorax risk, particularly with unusually deep or misplaced needle insertion. See the discussion of Spinal Accessory-I (3) in the previous chapter.

43. Superficial Peroneal (60.6%). This cutaneous nerve surfaces above the deep fascia to innervate the skin of the dorsum of the foot. It pierces the fascia immediately lateral to the tendon of the extensor digitorum longus in the anterior ankle, forming the acupoint. See Figure 5.1a and Figure 5.5a.

44. Sural-II (59.7%). This acupoint is 5 cm proximal to the Sural-I (10). See Figure 5.1b, Figure

5.5b, and the discussion of Sural-I (10) in the previous chapter.

45. Posterior Cutaneous of L3 (57.9%). This is the L3 equivalent of the Posterior Cutaneous of L2 (15) point discussed in the previous chapter. See Figure 5.1b, Figure 5.3b, Figure 5.4b, and the discussion of L2 (15) in the previous chapter.

46. Recurrent of Median (55.7%). This branch of the median nerve bifurcates from the main nerve in the palm of the hand and doubles back to enter the thenar muscles toward the base of the thumb, forming an acupoint. The location of the acupoint can be anywhere in the thenar eminence due to individual variations in the nerve but is usually found near the middle. See Figure 5.1a, Figure 5.4a, and the discussion in Chapter 3, including Figure 3.5a.

47. Posterior Cutaneous of T8 (55.2%). This is the T8 equivalent of the Posterior Cutaneous of T6 (21) acupoint, discussed in the previous chapter. See Figure 5.1b, Figure 5.3b, and Figure 5.4b.

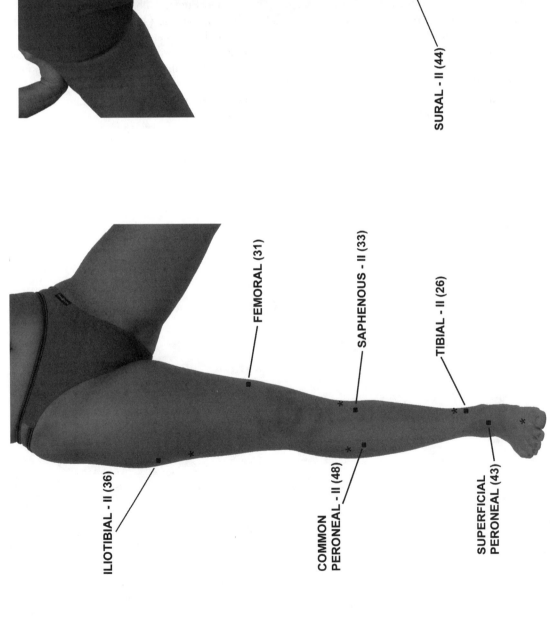

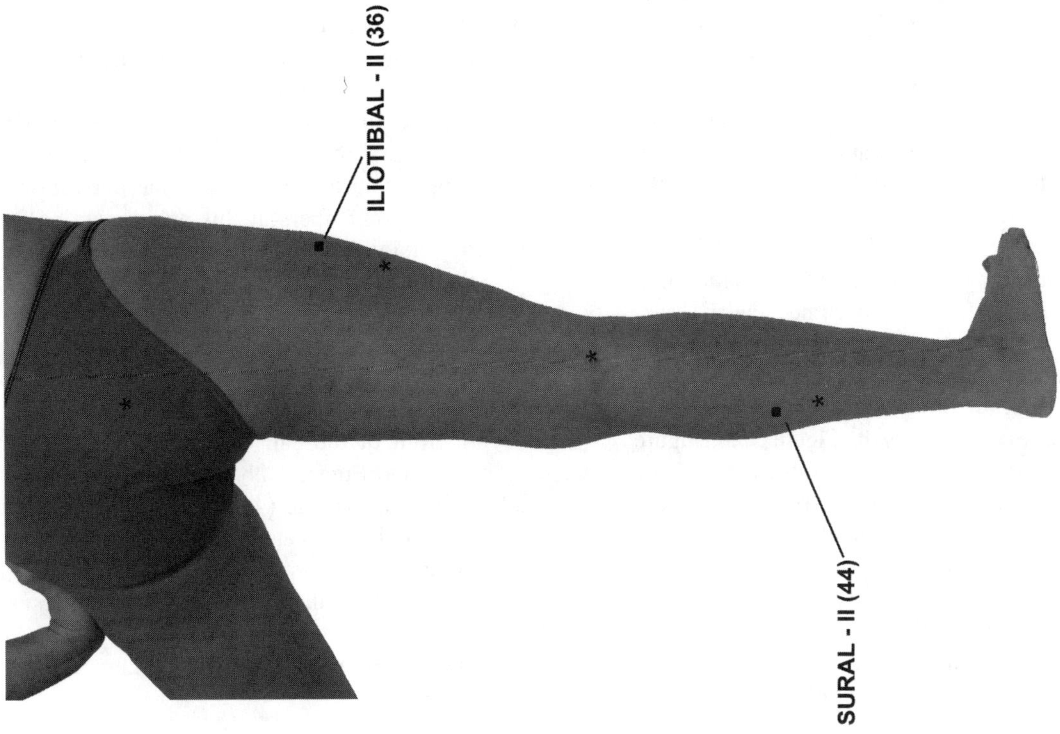

**FIGURE 5.5b** Secondary points of the lower extremity: posterior aspect.

**FIGURE 5.5a** Secondary points of the lower extremity: anterior aspect.

48. Common Peroneal-II (51.6%). This is about 3 cm distal and a little anterior to the Common Peroneal-I (24). See Figure 5.1a, Figure 5.5a, and the discussion of Common Peroneal-I (24) in the previous chapter.

49. Supraspinatus (50.2%). This point arising from a branch of the suprascapular nerve is similar to the Infraspinatus (8), its nerve entering the supraspinatus muscle from beneath. The supraspinatus muscle is thicker than the infraspinatus; therefore, the Infraspinatus point is more superficial and becomes tender earlier in the progression of pain. The neuromuscular attachment of the supraspinatus nerve is deeper than that of the infraspinatus and thus harder to palpate. See Figure 5.1b, Figure 5.2b, Figure 5.3b, Figure 5.4b, and the discussion of the Infraspinatus (8) point in the previous chapter. Dung's original work labeled this point the "Suprascapular-II."

50. Mental (49.8%). Innervated by the mandibular division of the fifth cranial nerve, this point is found over the mental foramen of the mandible, 2 to 3 cm below, and slightly medial to, the corner of the mouth. See Figure 5.1a and Figure 5.2a.

51. Superior Auricular (49.3%). This point is situated on the scalp at the position closest to the highest point of the helix of the ear. It is a neuromuscular attachment containing efferent fibers of the facial (VII) nerve to the superior auricular muscle. The derivation of the afferent fibers at this attachment is controversial because the facial nerve is not thought by many anatomists to contain afferent fibers. If the afferent fibers do not arise from the facial nerve, the most likely source is fibers from the mandibular division of the trigeminal (V) nerve progressing superiorly in front of the ear. See Figure 5.1a, Figure 5.2a, and Figure 5.2b.

52. Acromioclavicular (48.8%). The Acromioclavicular point is located superiorly over the acromioclavicular joint. The innervation of the acromioclavicular joint is essentially unknown. Possible sources include the lateral pectoral or medial pectoral nerves. See Figure 5.1a and Figure 5.4a.

# 6 The Tertiary Acupoints

## CONTENTS

## 6.1   INTRODUCTION

The tertiary points are generally less important systemically than the secondary points when acupuncture is considered as a treatment. In assessment, however, these points, if passive systemically, indicate a patient who has a relatively poor prognosis for pain management. As local points, these points may be frequently needled. The reader would benefit by reading through this chapter and locating the points on the figures, but memorization is generally not required. The following list is organized like those of the previous two chapters.

Figures throughout this text use a black circle as the symbol to depict tertiary points; the star symbol is used to designate primary points and the square symbol, secondary points.

## 6.2   TERTIARY ACUPOINTS

The tertiary acupoints are presented in the sequence of their becoming passive (Figure 6.1a and Figure 6.1b):

53. Transverse Cervical (48.8%). This acupoint is located at the anterior border of the sternocleidomastoid muscle at the same vertical level as the Cervical Plexus (28) acupoint (which is midway along the posterior sternocleidomastoid border). At the Transverse Cervical (53) acupoint, the nerve, coursing from the cervical plexus of which it is a branch, bifurcates into three or four subcutaneous bundles, each of which can form an acupoint. Needling in the anterior triangle of the neck should be undertaken with care not to puncture other important structures (particularly major arteries). See Figure 6.1a and Figure 6.2a.

54. Achilles (48.4%). These points are located on lateral and medial sides of the Achilles tendon about 2 or 3 cm proximal to its attachment at the calcaneus. They are innervated by the sural nerve, which passes deep to the lateral point. See Figure 6.1b, Figure 6.5b, and also Figure 3.3 in the chapter on pain quantification.

55. Upper Biceps Brachii (47.5%). This point is a neuromuscular attachment of the musculocutaneous nerve located in the mass of the biceps muscle approximately one third of the distance from the shoulder to the elbow along the anterior surface of the brachium. See Figure 6.1a, Figure 6.4a, and also Figure 3.4 in the chapter on pain quantification.

56. Inferolateral Malleolus (47.1%). This acupoint from the sural nerve appears just distal to the lateral malleolus. See Figure 6.1b and Figure 6.5b.

57. Inferomedial Malleolus (47.1%). This acupoint from the sural nerve appears just distal to the medial malleolus. See Figure 6.1b and Figure 6.5b.

58. Intercostobrachial (46.2%). This nerve from the lateral cutaneous branch of the anterior ramus of T2 is found in the chest wall approximately 7 to 8 cm inferior to the peak of the axilla in the mid-axillary line, where the nerve penetrates the second intercostal space. This nerve supplements the medial brachial cutaneous nerve in innervating the skin of the medial surface of the arm. In some individuals, this point is very sensitive, even if the individual's sensitivity is low. The intercostobrachial nerve has a curious, well-known relationship to the medial brachial cutaneous nerve in that usually one of the two is large and the other small, but which is the larger varies from individual to individual. This is unusual in that the two nerves have different derivations (see the derivation of the medial brachial cutaneous nerve from C8 and T1 in the discussion of the Medial Brachial

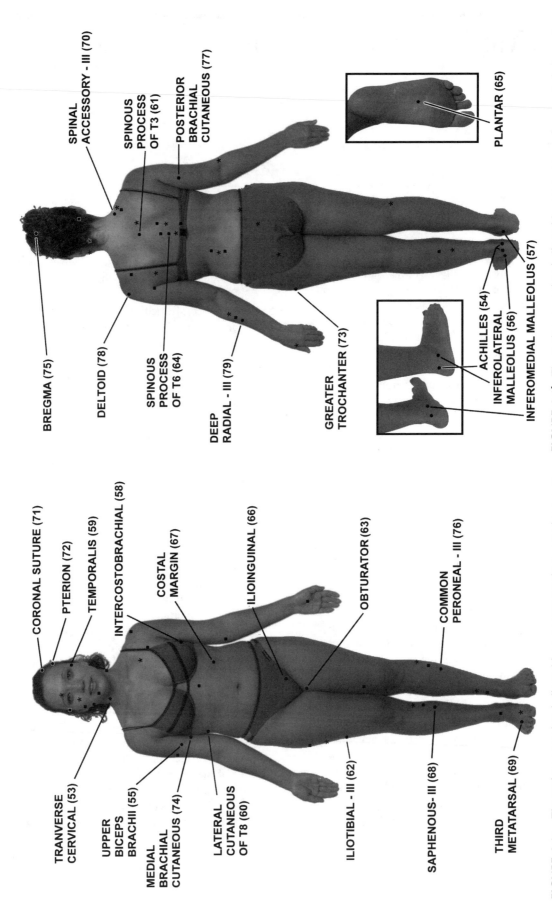

SPINAL ACCESSORY - III (70)
SPINOUS PROCESS OF T3 (61)
POSTERIOR BRACHIAL CUTANEOUS (77)
PLANTAR (65)
BREGMA (75)
DELTOID (78)
SPINOUS PROCESS OF T6 (64)
DEEP RADIAL - III (79)
GREATER TROCHANTER (73)
ACHILLES (54)
INFEROLATERAL MALLEOLUS (56)
INFEROMEDIAL MALLEOLUS (57)

**FIGURE 6.1b** The tertiary acupoints indicated by sequence numbers: posterior aspect.

CORONAL SUTURE (71)
PTERION (72)
TEMPORALIS (59)
INTERCOSTOBRACHIAL (58)
COSTAL MARGIN (67)
ILIOINGUINAL (66)
OBTURATOR (63)
COMMON PERONEAL - III (76)
TRANVERSE CERVICAL (53)
UPPER BICEPS BRACHII (55)
MEDIAL BRACHIAL CUTANEOUS (74)
LATERAL CUTANEOUS OF T8 (60)
ILIOTIBIAL - III (62)
SAPHENOUS- III (68)
THIRD METATARSAL (69)

**FIGURE 6.1a** The tertiary acupoints indicated by sequence numbers: anterior aspect.

Cutaneous (74) acupoint). The acupoint is a pneumothorax risk for needles placed more deeply than necessary. See Figure 6.1a, Figure 6.3a, Figure 6.4a, and Figure 6.4b.

59. Temporalis (6.2%). This neuromuscular attachment to the temporalis muscle originates from the mandibular division of the trigeminal nerve (the fifth cranial nerve). The nerve enters the temporalis muscle from deep within the temporal fossa. This acupoint is used occasionally for headache; infrequently, the adjacent temporal artery is pierced, creating a visible hematoma. See Figure 6.1a, Figure 6.2a, and Figure 6.2b.

60. Lateral Cutaneous of T8 (45.2%). This nerve is located in the mid-axillary line between the eighth and ninth ribs and derives from the anterior primary ramus of T8. Needles inserted deeply into this point can cause a pneumothorax. See Figure 6.1a, Figure 6.3a, and Figure 6.4b.

61. Spinous process of T3 (43.0%). This acupoint, like that of T7 discussed in Chapter 4, is formed by the ligamentum nuchae, an expansion of the supraspinous ligament that joins the tips of the spinous processes. T3 is located in the midpoint of a line joining the medial ends of the spines of the scapulae. See Figure 6.1b, Figure 6.2b, and Figure 6.3b, as well as discussion of the Spinous Process of T7 (20) acupoint discussed in Chapter 4.

62. Iliotibial-III (41.2%). This is approximately 6 to 7 cm distal to the Iliotibial-I (18) along the iliotibial tract. See Figure 6.1a, Figure 6.5a, and Figure 6.5b, as well as discussion of the Iliotibial-I (18) acupoint in Chapter 4.

63. Obturator (41.2%). This nerve from the lumbar spinal plexus, from the anterior primary rami of L2 through L4, leaves the pelvis through the obturator foramen to supply skin and muscles in the medial compartment of the thigh. Several points at the upper part of the medial thigh may be collectively designated as Obturator (63). In practice, these points are not often used because pain in this area is rare. The patients most commonly complaining of pain here have been injured in recreational sports such as speedboat racing and water skiing, pulling the thigh outward and damaging the attachments of the hamstring muscles (semimembranosus and semitendinosus) to the pelvic bone. See Figure 6.1a, Figure 6.5a, and Figure 6.5b.

64. Spinous Process of T6 (37.6%). This is the T6 equivalent of the Spinous Process of T7 (20) acupoint, discussed in Chapter 4. See Figure 6.1b, Figure 6.2b, and Figure 6.3b.

65. Plantar (36.7%). This is derived from the cutaneous terminal branch of the tibial nerve. Actually, several plantar points can form over the plantar surface of the foot, the most common of which is 1 to 2 cm medial to the middle of its plantar surface. See Figures 6.1b and 6.5b.

66. Ilioinguinal (35.8%). This point is derived from the middle branch of the anterior primary ramus of L1. It courses along the inside of the posterior abdominal wall to the superficial inguinal ring where it becomes superficial and forms an acupoint. The point is superficial to the inguinal ring along the inguinal ligament immediately lateral to the tendon of the pectineal muscle at the superior border of the femoral triangle. This is not an important point therapeutically, but is found to be passive in those older patients who have had longstanding back pain. See Figure 6.1a, Figure 6.3a, Figure 6.4a, and Figure 6.5a.

67. Costal Margin (35.3%). This point is slightly lateral to the mid-clavicular line just inferior to the 10th rib. This is the anterior cutaneous nerve of T6. See Figure 6.1a, Figure 6.3a, and Figure 6.4a.

68. Saphenous-III (34.4%). This is approximately 2 to 3 cm distal to the Saphenous-II (33) acupoint. See Figure 6.1a and Figure 6.5a, a well as the discussion of the Saphenous-I (4) acupoint in Chapter 4.

69. Third Metatarsal (33.0%). This terminal branch of the common peroneal nerve (from the lateral side of the sciatic nerve) is located over the distal end of the third metatarsal bone. See Figure 6.1a and Figure 6.5a.

70. Spinal Accessory-III (32.6%). Please refer to the discussion of Spinal Accessory-II (42) in the previous chapter. If a third point is found in the general area of Spinal Accessory-I (3), then it is designated Spinal Accessory-III and its presence may be significant in the individual's pain quantification or it may indicate a local problem. See Figure 6.1b, Figure 6.2b, Figure 6.3b, and Figure 6.4b.

71. Coronal Suture (32.1%). This acupoint is innervated by the ophthalmic division of the trigeminal nerve (fifth cranial nerve) and is located along the suture approximately 6 cm inferior to the Bregma (75). See Figure 6.1a and Figure 6.2a.

72. Pterion (32.1%). This acupoint is located at the site of the anterolateral fontanelle, about 3 cm superior to the highest point of the helix of the ear. The pterion receives its innervation from the supraorbital and auriculotemporal nerves. See Figure 6.1a and Figure 6.2a.

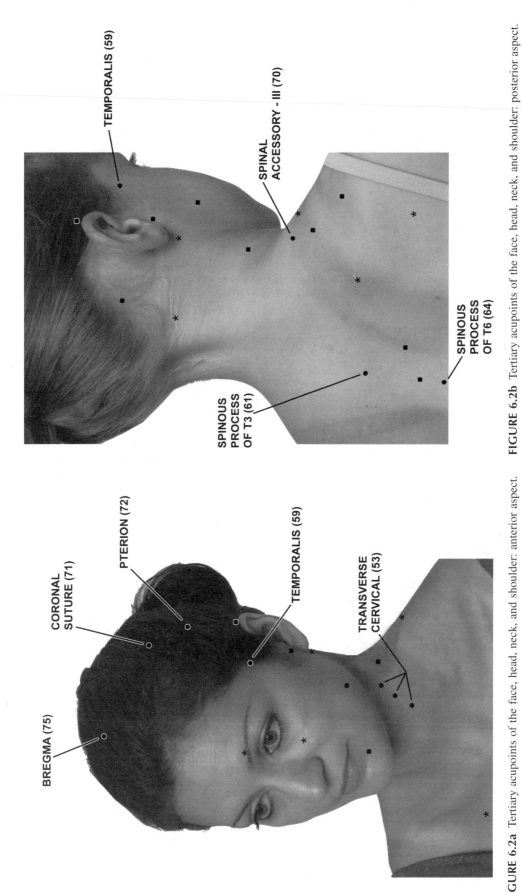

**FIGURE 6.2b** Tertiary acupoints of the face, head, neck, and shoulder: posterior aspect.

**FIGURE 6.2a** Tertiary acupoints of the face, head, neck, and shoulder: anterior aspect.

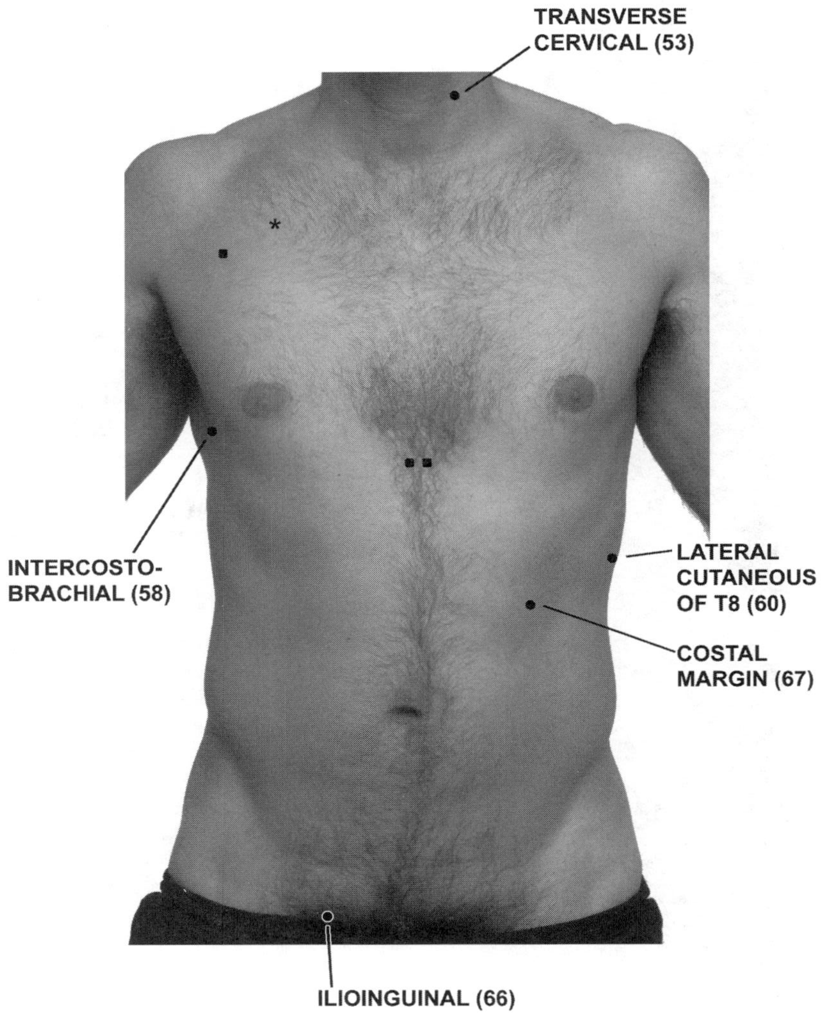

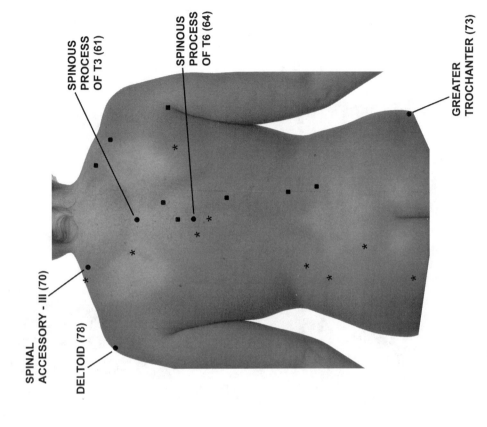

**FIGURE 6.3b** Tertiary acupoints of the thorax and abdomen: posterior aspect.

**FIGURE 6.3a** Tertiary acupoints of the thorax and abdomen: anterior aspect.

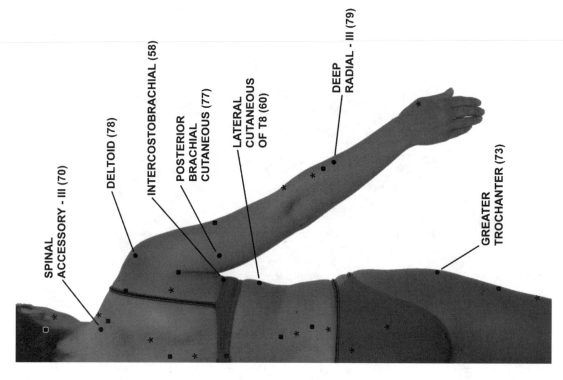

**FIGURE 6.4b** Tertiary acupoints of the upper extremity: posterior aspect.

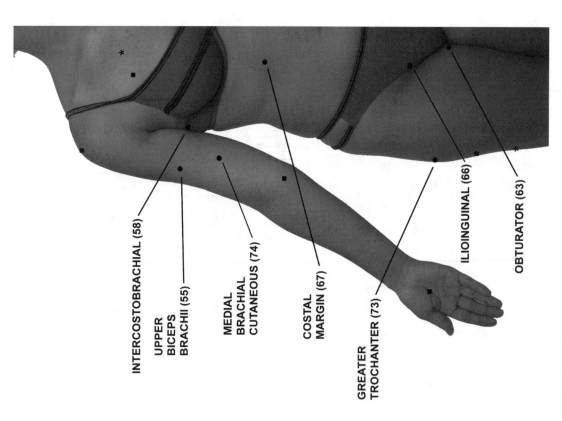

**FIGURE 6.4a** Tertiary acupoints of the upper extremity: anterior aspect.

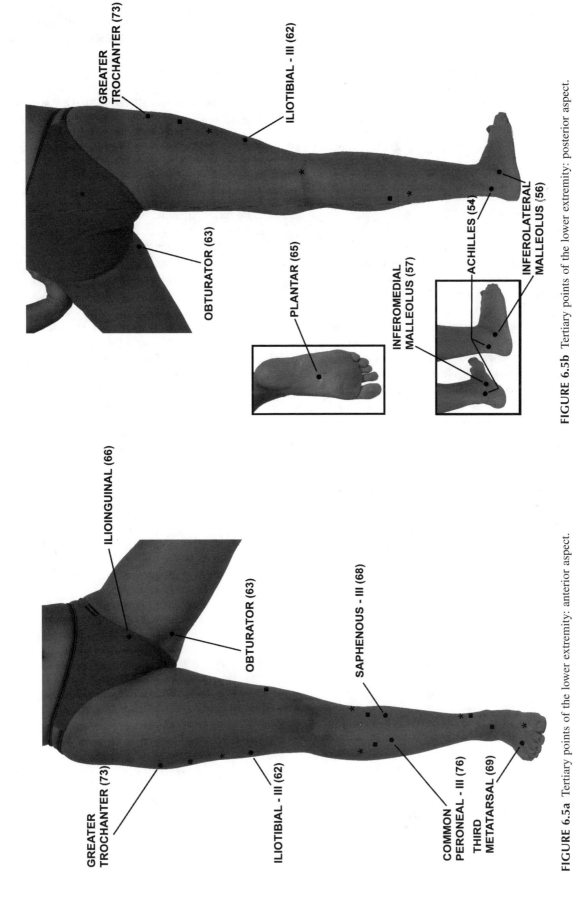

**FIGURE 6.5b**  Tertiary points of the lower extremity: posterior aspect.

**FIGURE 6.5a**  Tertiary points of the lower extremity: anterior aspect.

GREATER TROCHANTER (73)

ILIOTIBIAL - III (62)

OBTURATOR (63)

PLANTAR (65)

INFEROMEDIAL MALLEOLUS (57)

ACHILLES (54)

INFEROLATERAL MALLEOLUS (56)

ILIOINGUINAL (66)

OBTURATOR (63)

SAPHENOUS - III (68)

GREATER TROCHANTER (73)

ILIOTIBIAL - III (62)

COMMON PERONEAL - III (76)

THIRD METATARSAL (69)

73. Greater Trochanter (31.7%). This point is quite easy to palpate over the greater trochanter of the femur. No conspicuous nerve is located in this area, and pain is most likely due to inflammation of the bursa overlying the bone. As many as a half-dozen points may overlay the greater trochanter. See Figure 6.1b, Figure 6.3b, Figure 6.4a, Figure 6.4b, Figure 6.5a, and Figure 6.5b.

74. Medial Brachial Cutaneous (31.2%). This nerve, derived from C8 and T1, penetrates the deep fascia at the midpoint of the line connecting the axillary pit and the medial epicondyle of the humerus. Before emerging from the deep fascia, the medial brachial cutaneous nerve is situated deep inside the medial side of the arm in a space known as the neurovascular compartment of the brachium. Although four big nerve trunks are inside the compartment, only one acupoint is in this relatively large area in the medial surface of the arm because all the other nerve trunks are situated rather deeply. The Medial Brachial Cutaneous point is formed as the nerve branches from the ulnar nerve and emerges from the deep fascia to become superficial. See the discussion of the Intercostobrachial (58) point regarding the curious relationship between the two nerves and also Figure 6.1a and Figure 6.4a.

75. Bregma (30.3%). Suture lines are areas in which the individual bones of the skull join; these are likely to form acupoints, especially in patients with chronic headaches. One such point is the bregma, located at the juncture of the coronal and sagittal sutures. This point is located at the site of the cartilaginous anterior fontanelle in infants. This fontanelle is the last to close, which may account for the fact that skin over the bregma has richer innervation than the surrounding bony skull. See Figure 6.1b and Figure 6.2a.

76. Common Peroneal-III (29.4%). This acupoint is approximately 3 cm distal to the Common Peroneal-II (48) along the lateral border of the tibia. It is slightly proximal to the midpoint of the length of the tibia. See Figure 6.1a and Figure 6.5a, as well as the discussion of Common Peroneal-I (24) in Chapter 4.

77. Posterior Brachial Cutaneous (28.5%). This nerve is a branch of the radial nerve. Like the acupoints of other cutaneous nerves, the Posterior Brachial Cutaneous point is formed at the location at which the nerve emerges from the deep fascia. This is not an important point and is not used clinically very often. It is located midway along the posterior surface of the brachium. See Figure 6.1b and Figure 6.4b.

78. Deltoid (28.5%). This acupoint develops from one of several potential points innervated by the axillary nerve and is located along the attachment of the deltoid muscle to the acromion process of the scapula. See Figure 6.1b, Figure 6.3b, and Figure 6.4b.

79. Deep Radial-III (27.7%). This point is approximately 2 to 3 cm distal to the Deep Radial-II (29). See Figure 6.1b and Figure 6.4b, Figure 3.2a in the chapter on pain quantification, and the discussion of Deep Radial-I (1) in Chapter 4.

# 7 The Nonspecific Acupoints

## CONTENTS

## 7.1 INTRODUCTION

Systemically, the nonspecific acupoints are unimportant other than as indicators of patients with very poor prognoses. Their systemic presence suggests a diagnosis of fibromyalgia with diffuse sensitivity of nociceptive tissue throughout the body. Locally, they are useful as tender points around an injury that will respond to needles.

Sequence numbers assigned to the nonspecific points are somewhat arbitrary because individuals vary so much. They are assigned here to provide a reference framework for future research. Also, readers of Dung's earlier text, *Anatomical Acupuncture*, will note that points 87 through 112 have been renumbered to reflect the insertion of T1 and T9 in the sequence. Many of these points derive from nerves that have been poorly studied, so the following discussions of these derivations are somewhat speculative. The list in this chapter is included only for completeness; the reader may want to read through this chapter and locate the points, but it is not essential to do so. The clinician, however, when faced with an unfamiliar local problem, may want to examine the figure here to determine the local points in the anatomical area that would be appropriate for needling.

Figures throughout this text use a white circle as the symbol to depict nonspecific points; recall that the star symbol is used to designate primary points; the square symbol, secondary points; and the black circle, tertiary points.

## 7.2 NONSPECIFIC ACUPOINTS

The nonspecific acupoints are presented in the sequence of their becoming passive (Figure 7.1a and Figure 7.1b):

80. Intermediate Supraclavicular (27.6%). The supraclavicular nerves (lateral, intermediate, and medial) derive from C3 and C4 and become superficial just above the clavicle to supply skin over the clavicle, upper thorax, and upper shoulder. The Intermediate Supraclavicular is a pair of acupoints, one located at the superior border of the clavicle at its midpoint and the other just below the first, below the clavicle. The other two related acupoints are the Medial Supraclavicular (85) and the Lateral Supraclavicular (86), discussed later. See Figure 7.1a (depicting only the superior point), Figure 7.2a, Figure 7.3a, and Figure 7.4a.

81. Fifth Metatarsal (27.1%). This acupoint is located on the lateral side of the head of the fifth metatarsal bone (just proximal to the metatarsophalangeal joint). This cutaneous area is innervated by terminal branches of the sural nerve. See Figure 7.1a, Figure 7.1b, Figure 7.5a, and Figure 7.5b.

82. Medial Sural (26.2%). This point at a bifurcation of the medial sural (or "crural") nerve is located approximately 5 cm distal to the popliteal fossa in the middle of the medial head of the gastrocnemius muscle. See Figure 7.1b and Figure 7.5b.

83. Zygomaticofacial (24.9%). This point is formed by the zygomaticofacial nerve, a cutaneous branch of the maxillary division of the trigeminal nerve (V) that emerges superficially through the zygomaticofacial foramen located on the zygomatic bone. As an individual ages, this foramen becomes smaller and eventually disappears; this is a possible reason that some headaches tend to diminish with age. See Figure 7.1a and Figure 7.2a.

84. Saphenous-N (23.1%). This is a nonspecific point at the midpoint of the posterior border of the tibia. See also discussions of the Saphenous-I (4), Saphenous-II (33), and the Saphenous-III (68) in Chapter 4 through Chapter 6, respectively. See Figure 7.1a and Figure 7.5a.

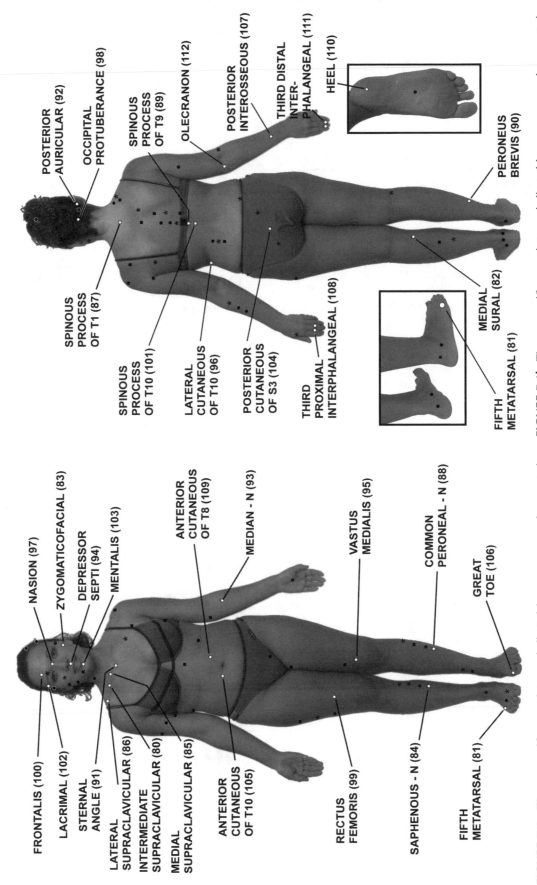

**FIGURE 7.1b** The nonspecific acupoints are indicated by sequence numbers: posterior aspect.

**FIGURE 7.1a** The nonspecific acupoints are indicated by sequence numbers: anterior aspect.

85. Medial Supraclavicular (21.7%). Like the intermediate supraclavicular discussed previously, the medial supraclavicular nerve is a terminal branch of the supraclavicular nerve. Actually two Medial Supraclavicular acupoints are approximately 2 to 3 cm lateral to the medial end of the clavicle on the superior and inferior clavicular borders. See Figure 7.1a (depicting only the superior point), Figure 7.2a, and Figure 7.3a.

86. Lateral Supraclavicular (19.9%). Similar to the intermediate supraclavicular and the medial supraclavicular nerves, this terminal branch of the supraclavicular nerve forms acupoints approximately 4 cm medial to the distal end of the clavicle along its superior and inferior borders. See Figure 7.1a (depicting only the superior point), Figure 7.2a, Figure 7.3a, and Figure 7.4a.

87. Spinous Process of T1 (19.2%). This acupoint, like that of T7 discussed in Chapter 4, is formed by the ligamentum nuchae, an expansion of the supraspinous ligament that joins the tips of the spinous processes. The spinous process of T1 is located about 1 to 2 cm inferior to the vertebral prominence that is the spinous process of the seventh cervical vertebra. See Figure 7.1b, Figure 7.2b, and Figure 7.3b, as well as the discussion in Chapter 4 of the Spinous Process of T7 (20) acupoint.

88. Common Peroneal-N (18.6%). This point is on the lateral tibial border at the midpoint of its length and is the last point of the chain of common peroneal points that include the Common Peroneal-I (24), Common Peroneal-II (48), and Common Peroneal-III (76). See Figure 7.1a, Figure 7.5a, and the discussion of companion acupoints along the common peroneal nerve in Chapter 2 through Chapter 4.

89. Spinous Process of T9 (17.8%). This acupoint, as previously stated in the discussion of T7 in Chapter 4 and T1 (87) previously, is formed by the ligamentum nuchae, an expansion of the supraspinous ligament that joins the tips of the spinous processes. The spinous process of T9 is two processes below that of T7; the latter is located in the midpoint of a line connecting the inferior angles of the scapulae. See Figure 7.1b, Figure 7.3b, and the discussion in Chapter 4 of the Spinous Process of T7 (20) acupoint.

90. Peroneus Brevis (17.6%). This acupoint probably is derived from a muscular branch of the common peroneal nerve where it enters the peroneus brevis muscle approximately three quarters of the length of the fibula from knee to ankle over lateral surface of the bone. The precise derivation of this minor point is unknown. See Figure 7.1b, Figure 7.5a, and Figure 7.5b.

91. Sternal Angle (16.7%). As its name implies, this point is located at the sternal angle between the manubrium and sternal body. It probably derives from the medial supraclavicular nerve. Note that another useful but unnumbered point is in the midline of the sternal notch. See Figure 7.1a and Figure 7.3a.

92. Posterior Auricular (15.8%). This acupoint is located immediately behind the center of the ear in the posterior auricular muscle, at the crease where the skin of the ear meets the scalp. Its efferent fibers probably originate from a branch of the facial nerve and its afferent fibers may originate from the mandibular branch of the trigeminal nerve. See Figure 7.1b and Figure 7.2b.

93. Median-N (15.4%). The median nerve in the forearm may form as many as four acupoints along its course and this one is located most proximally of the four. It is approximately 0.5 cm on the radial side of a line from the middle of the cubital fossa to the middle of the volar aspect of the wrist, approximately 3 cm from the cubital fossa. See Figure 7.1a and Figure 7.4a.

94. Depressor Septi (14.5%). In the mid-sagittal line immediately below the nose, a passive point can occur superficially on the depressor septi muscle. It is innervated by the maxillary division of the trigeminal nerve. See Figure 7.1a and Figure 7.2a.

95. Vastus Medialis (12.7%). The Vastus Medialis acupoint is just superior to the anterior surface of the medial epicondyle of the femur. The Vastus Lateralis point, an unnumbered point in Dung's original studies, is located just superior to the anterior surface of the lateral epicondyle of the femur and seems to be roughly equivalent to the Vastus Medialis point. See Figure 7.1a and Figure 7.5a for the numbered point.

96. Lateral Cutaneous of T10 (11.8%). The lateral cutaneous nerves are terminal branches of the thoracic spinal nerves. They circle the torso to emerge along the mid-axillary line. The Lateral Cutaneous of T10 emerges at the level of the 10th rib. See Figure 7.1b, Figure 7.3b, and Figure 7.4b.

97. Nasion (10.9%). The nasion is defined as the point where the internasal and frontonasal sutures meet. The Nasion acupoint can become passive even if the patient does not have headaches. If a patient has tenderness at this point and is a headache sufferer, the headaches will

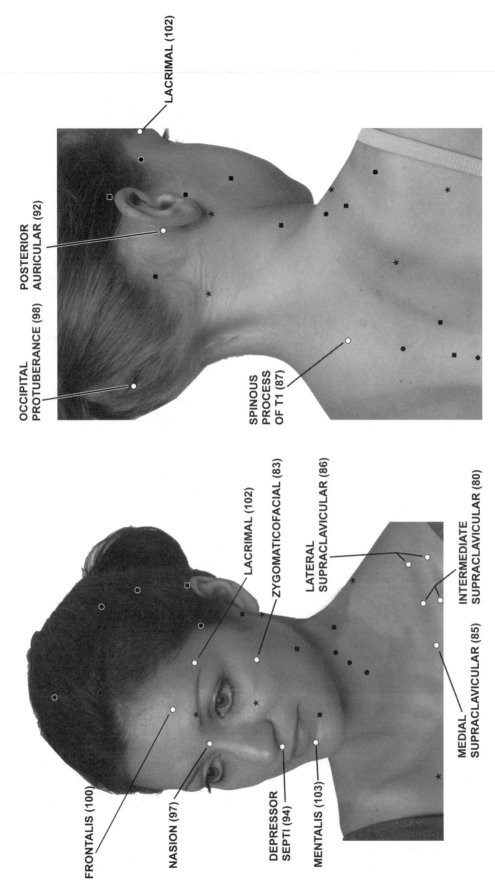

**FIGURE 7.2b** Nonspecific acupoints of the face, head, neck, and shoulder: posterior aspect.

**FIGURE 7.2a** Nonspecific acupoints of the face, head, neck, and shoulder: anterior aspect.

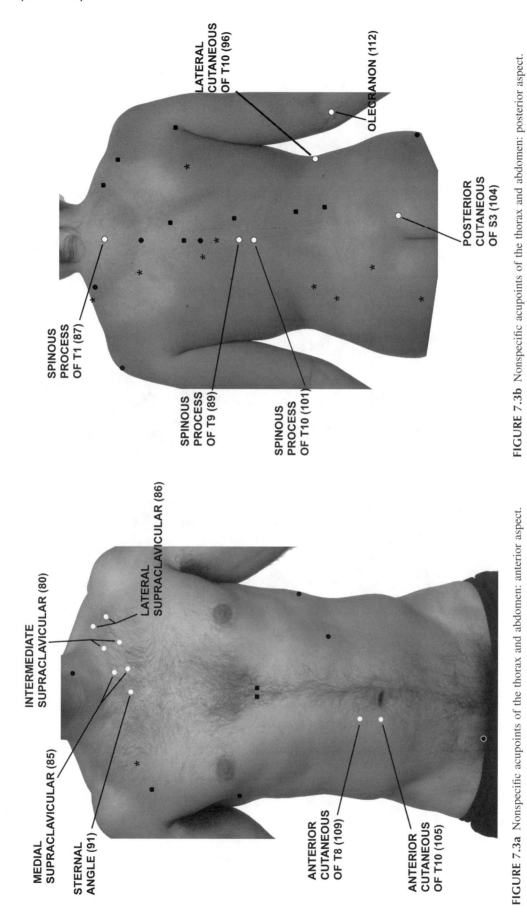

**FIGURE 7.3b** Nonspecific acupoints of the thorax and abdomen: posterior aspect.

**FIGURE 7.3a** Nonspecific acupoints of the thorax and abdomen: anterior aspect.

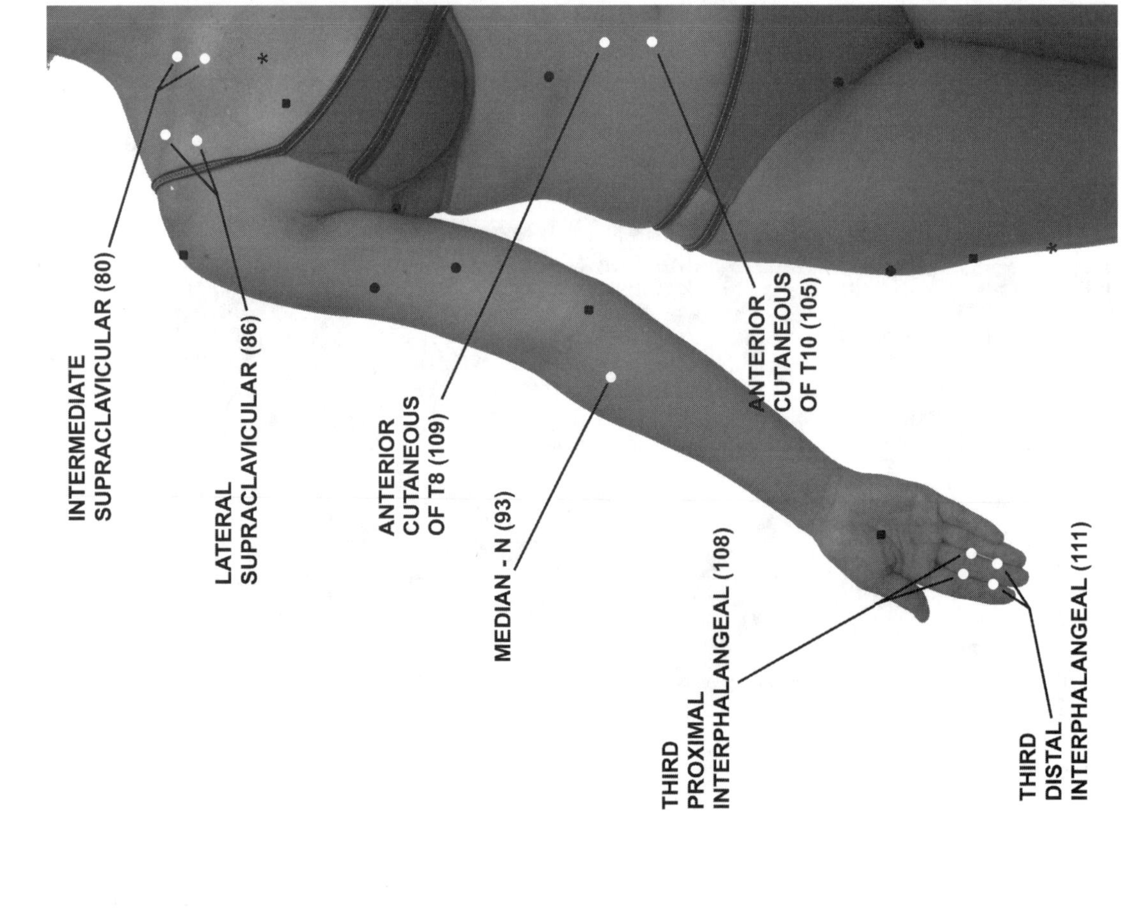

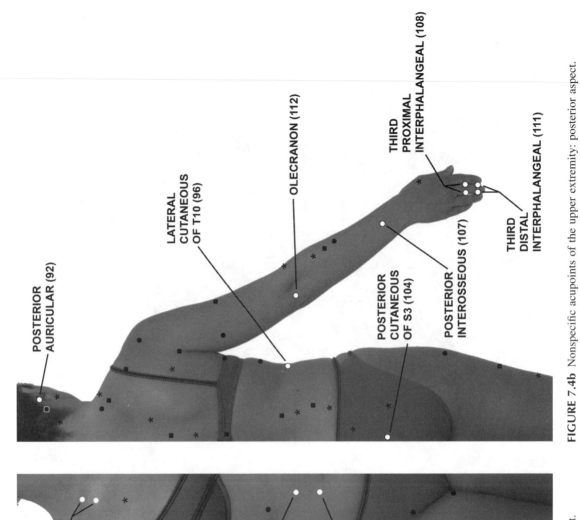

**FIGURE 7.4b** Nonspecific acupoints of the upper extremity: posterior aspect.

**FIGURE 7.4a** Nonspecific acupoints of the upper extremity: anterior aspect.

POSTERIOR AURICULAR (92)

LATERAL CUTANEOUS OF T10 (96)

OLECRANON (112)

THIRD PROXIMAL INTERPHALANGEAL (108)

POSTERIOR CUTANEOUS OF S3 (104)

POSTERIOR INTEROSSEOUS (107)

THIRD DISTAL INTERPHALANGEAL (111)

INTERMEDIATE SUPRACLAVICULAR (80)

LATERAL SUPRACLAVICULAR (86)

ANTERIOR CUTANEOUS OF T8 (109)

MEDIAN - N (93)

THIRD PROXIMAL INTERPHALANGEAL (108)

THIRD DISTAL INTERPHALANGEAL (111)

ANTERIOR CUTANEOUS OF T10 (105)

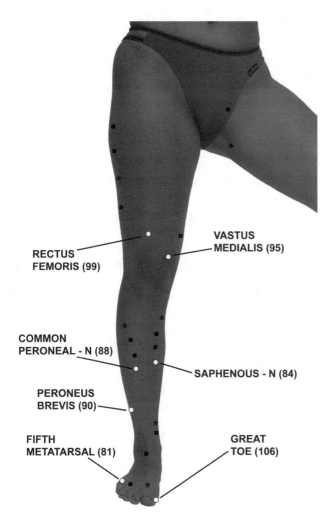

FIGURE 7.5a Nonspecific points of the lower extremity: anterior aspect.

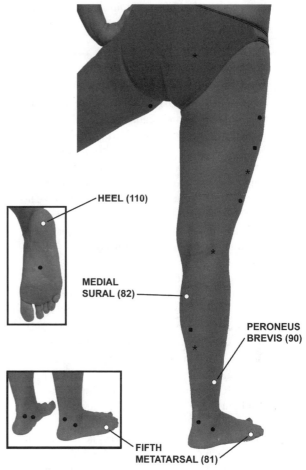

FIGURE 7.5b Nonspecific points of the lower extremity: posterior aspect.

be very difficult to manage. This point is most likely innervated by a tiny branch of the supraorbital nerve from the ophthalmic division of the trigeminal nerve. See Figure 7.1a and Figure 7.2a.

98. Occipital Protuberance (9.5%). The Occipital Protuberance can become tender on a few headache patients; this point is very easy to locate and detect. Like the Nasion (97) acupoint, if this point is passive, it has poor prognostic significance for headache sufferers. It may originate from the lesser or greater occipital nerves (or both); the anatomy of these tiny nerves is poorly understood. See Figure 7.1b and Figure 7.2b.

99. Rectus Femoris (9.0%). Damage or injury to the rectus femoris muscle, e.g., an automobile accident in which a thigh is crushed, can produce a passive acupoint on the distal end of the muscle about 7 or 8 cm superior to the middle of the patella. This area is innervated by the femoral nerve and its branches. See Figure 7.1a and Figure 7.5a.

100. Frontalis (8.1%). This acupoint may appear at the center of the frontalis muscle on the forehead, particularly in chronic headache patients. This is about 3 cm superior and slightly lateral to the Supraorbital (23) acupoint. It receives its efferent fibers from the facial (VII) nerve and its afferent fibers from the supraorbital nerve (from the ophthalmic division of the trigeminal nerve). See Figure 7.1a and Figure 7.2a.

101. Spinous Process of T10 (7.6%). The location on the tip of the spinal process of the 10th thoracic vertebrae can become an acupoint. See the preceding discussion of the Spinous Process of T1 (87), Figure 7.1b, and Figure 7.3b.

102. Lacrimal (7.2%). Small twigs of the lacrimal nerve become cutaneous over the lateral brim of the orbit where a passive acupoint can emerge. This acupoint is about 1 cm superior to the lateral end of the eyebrow. See Figure 7.1a, Figure 7.2a, and Figure 7.2b.

103. Mentalis (6.8%). This acupoint is named Mentalis because of its location between mentalis muscles under the lower lip. It is found in the midline about 5 mm below the vermilion line of the lip. It derives from mental nerve, a branch of the inferior alveolar nerve, itself a branch of the mandibular division of the trigeminal nerve. See Figure 7.1a and Figure 7.2a.

104. Posterior Cutaneous of S3 (6.3%). This acupoint is formed by the posterior cutaneous branch of the posterior primary ramus of the third sacral spinal nerve and is found about 5 cm superior to the tip of the coccyx and 3 cm lateral to the midline. This acupoint is often tender in a patient with a coccyx injury. See Figure 7.1b, Figure 7.3b, and Figure 7.4b.

105. Anterior Cutaneous of T10 (5.9%). The terminal branches of the anterior cutaneous nerves from the thoracic spinal nerves can form acupoints where the branches penetrate the deep fascia, approximately 2 to 4 cm on either side of the sternal line from the upper sternum to the lower abdomen. The T10 point and the T8 point are the most likely of these to become tender. This point is about 3 to 4 cm lateral to umbilicus. See Figure 7.1a, Figure 7.3a, and Figure 7.4a.

106. Great Toe (5.4%). A passive acupoint can appear on the medial area between the proximal and distal phalanges of the first or big toe, more or less over the interphalangeal joint. It probably is derived from the deep peroneal (also called "fibular" in some texts) or medial plantar nerves. See Figure 7.1a and Figure 7.5a.

107. Posterior Interosseous (5.0%). The posterior interosseous nerve is a terminal branch of deep radial nerve. This branch runs posteriorly on the interosseous membrane connecting the ulna and radius and innervates the wrist joint. The acupoint is located about 4 cm proximal to the middle of the dorsal crease of the wrist. See Figure 7.1b and Figure 7.4b.

108. Third Proximal Interphalangeal (4.0%). Although there is some individual variation, on the dorsal aspect of the hand the ulnar side is typically innervated by the ulnar nerve and the radial side is innervated by the superficial radial nerve. The palmar side is innervated primarily by the median nerve medially and the ulnar nerve for the little finger and ulnar side of the ring finger. All the cutaneous nerves to the fingers are derived from these three nerves and are called proper digital nerves. These nerves run down the radial and ulnar sides of the digits — four nerves around each joint (proximal inter-

phalangeal and distal interphalangeal): two on the radial side (one palmar and one dorsal); and the other two on the ulnar side (again, one palmar and one dorsal). The dorsal nerves are bigger and thus more important. These nerves contribute to the formation of four acupoints around each joint: two on the radial and ulnar sides of the joint and two on the palmar and dorsal sides of the joint.

The proximal interphalangeal joint is more likely to be involved in rheumatoid arthritis and the distal one in osteoarthritis. The Third Proximal Interphalangeal (108) acupoint refers to the middle finger and the radial and ulnar sides of its joint (which are not distinguished because they are usually palpated together by squeezing the joint). There are similar points around the distal joint, such as the Third Distal Interphalangeal (111). A good rule of thumb for either joint (in any of the digits, for that matter) is that if the palmar and dorsal sides of the joint are tender, the pain will be nearly impossible to manage with acupuncture, but if only the radial and ulnar sides are involved, acupuncture has a good chance of helping. If none of the four acupoints around the joint is tender (passive), pain in the joint will be exceedingly easy to manage with needles in the primary points without the need to place needles around the joint. See Figure 7.1b, Figure 7.4a, and Figure 7.4b.

109. Anterior Cutaneous of T8 (3.6%). See the preceding discussion of the Anterior Cutaneous of T10 (105). The T8 point is located midway between the lower rib border and the level of the umbilicus. See Figure 7.1a, Figure 7.3a, and Figure 7.4a.

110. Heel (3.2%). No named branch of any nerve goes to the heel of the foot. The area receives innervation from sural and plantar nerves. Passive acupoints can frequently appear in the heels of patients with podiatric problems. This point is located in the middle of the plantar surface of the calcaneus. See Figure 7.1b and Figure 7.5b.

111. Third Distal Interphalangeal (2.7%). See the preceding discussion of the Third Proximal Interphalangeal (108) and Figure 7.1b, Figure 7.4a, and Figure 7.4b.

112. Olecranon (1.4%). The proximal end of the ulna on the posterior side of the elbow is called the olecranon. The point is very easy to palpate and locate. Innervation of this acupoint may be derived from the medial brachial cutaneous nerve (from the medial cord of the brachial

plexus) or the posterior antebrachial cutaneous (from the radial nerve deriving from the posterior cord of the brachial plexus). See Figure 7.1b, Figure 7.3b, and Figure 7.4b.

## REFERENCES

1. Dung, H.C. *Anatomical Acupuncture*. Antarctic Press, San Antonio, 1997.

# 8 The Treatment Plan

## CONTENTS

## 8.1  OVERVIEW OF A COURSE OF THERAPY

The planning of a course of therapy is quite simple. In the ideal situation, treatment sessions are given in groups of three or four; the sessions are 2 to 3 days apart because this timing seems to be most efficacious and least likely to produce unpleasant side effects. After three or four sessions, the patient is given a week's rest without treatment and is then interviewed to determine what response has been achieved. At that point, another three to four sessions can be started or, if the problem is resolved, the response is unsatisfactory, or the patient expresses unwillingness to continue the course of treatment, acupuncture can be terminated in favor of other modalities. If the response is as expected given the patient's pain quantification and the patient wants to continue, the process is simply repeated as many times as necessary: three or four treatments over the course of a week, a week's rest, and reevaluation. These groups of three or four sessions over the course of about a week will be called *treatment series* in this text.

Sometimes, because of travel time, work issues, and other patient factors, it is impractical to follow the ideal course of therapy. Although the practitioner can afford to be flexible, in these instances the patient should be cautioned about the consequences of an altered schedule. If treatment sessions are too close together, the patient is likely to experience increased aching, regional pain, or other side effects (described in the next chapter); if they are too far apart, the patient may have a less efficacious response. The purpose of the week's rest is to allow a delayed response to develop: the patient may notice no difference for several days after completing the treatment series, only to experience a dramatic response as much as 7 to 10 days later.

If the patient has not had acupuncture within the last year, he or she is likely to experience a latent reaction (flare-up of pain, drowsiness or sleepiness, or parasympa-

thetic enhancement) after the first session. These are described more fully in the next chapter. The extent of this reaction is roughly proportional to the number of needles used in the session, so few needles should be used in the first session (no more than 20 to 25) and the patient should be warned about the possibility of reaction. Typically, these reactions last a few hours to a day at most. A strong reaction, although distressing to the patient, is reassuring to the clinician because it indicates a greater eventual likelihood of success with acupuncture. This is an illustration of an important rule: any physiologic reaction to acupuncture, whether immediate or delayed, or initially perceived as positive or negative, indicates a greater likelihood of eventual success.

## 8.2  PATIENT POSITIONING

Figure 8.1 through Figure 8.4 show the commonly used positions: prone, supine, side, and sitting. Several simple, but often contradictory, principles should be kept in mind. First, the clinician needs to be able to access the area of concern. If the patient is being treated for headaches, the accessibility of the head is especially important and a sitting position is often used; for neck and shoulder pain, a prone position is more appropriate. However, the position should be varied from session to session because points that are needled every session are more likely to become bruised and sore and develop hematomas. (Another consideration is that more acupoints are accessible when the patient is in the prone position, so if a patient who has never had acupuncture is started in the prone position, more restraint is called for.)

Also, the clinician may want to consider whether the first-time patient should be in a position in which he or she can see the needles as they are inserted; if the patient is particularly anxious about needles, a prone position may be a better way to begin. Another approach would be to

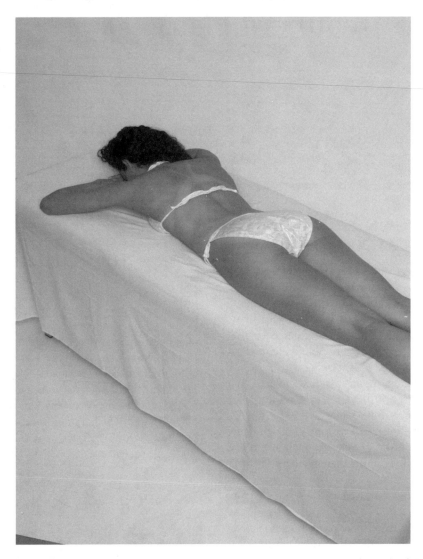

**FIGURE 8.1** The prone position for acupuncture. Although not shown, it is customary to pull the back of the patient's underwear down far enough to expose the inferior gluteal (16) acupoints. Male and female patients seem comfortable with this approach. Brassieres do not typically need to be removed unless they have a particularly wide strap across the back; in that case they can usually simply be unfastened. Also, lying on an examining table with a doughnut-shaped extension for the face is more comfortable for the patient than lying in the position shown.

use an "eye pillow"* or other blindfolding technique, along with music or other distractions. The sitting position has its own particular concern: syncope is a frequent reaction to needles administered in this position. Having the patient put his or her head down on an examining table (see Figure 8.4) seems to minimize the likelihood of this reaction. One method of doing this involves placing the required needles on the anterior surface of the body (especially the face) and then gently bending the patient over into the head-down position depicted in Figure 8.4 for placement of the dorsal needles. The side position is used

in some circumstances described in later chapters; when the patient is on the left side, the right leg should come over the left and rest on the table, bringing the patient's center of gravity toward the front of the body.

Another consideration is room temperature. Often patients complain of being too cold while waiting for the practitioner to enter the room to place the needles, but once the needles are placed, most patients feel warm immediately. Ideally, then, the patient should not undress and be put into position until the practitioner is almost ready to place the needles. A blanket should be available.

The preferred sequence of positions for different conditions is discussed in the chapters that discuss those conditions. As an example, however, consider a headache patient. This patient might be treated face up the first

---

* An "eye pillow" is a small cloth bag filled with grain or some lightweight pellets that can be placed over the eyes of a supine patient to shut out light and other visual stimulation. They are often found for sale in stores catering to frequent travelers and wilderness trekkers.

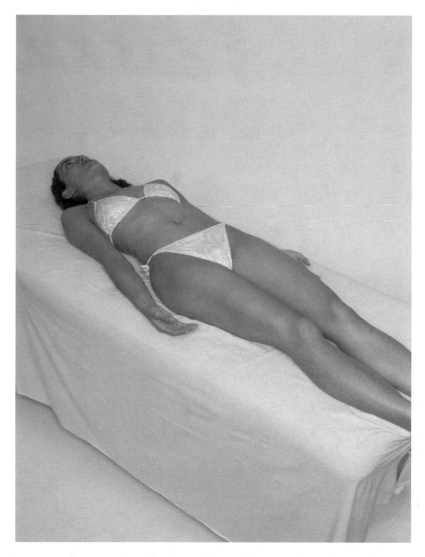

**FIGURE 8.2** The supine position for acupuncture. Another option for the arms and hands, especially on narrow tables, is for the patient to fold them across the abdomen.

session, face down the next, and sitting the third. If the patient has not been needled before, fewer needles might be inserted the first session. If a first-time patient has an aversion to needles, a face-down position may be more appropriate for the first session with a small number of needles placed (maybe just those in the head and neck), followed by face up the second session, and sitting the third. A first-time patient with neck and shoulder pain might be treated prone the first session, with needles placed only in the head and neck region and possibly the upper back. Then, in the second session, a supine position would be used with the normal number of needles placed; finally, in the third session, after the prospect of a latent reaction is minimized, the patient would be positioned face down and an increased number of points needled. Alternatively, four treatment sessions could be used in the treatment series: the first, face down with only a few needles; the second, face down with more

needles being placed; the third, supine; and the fourth, prone again.

The clinician should maintain some flexibility in applying these considerations. In general, there is a lot of room for variation in performing acupuncture without any great loss in efficacy.

## 8.3 GENERAL NEEDLE PLACEMENT

Needles are placed into tender acupoints. A patient with a pain sensitivity of one will have at most eight systemic points tender or passive on each half of the body (refer to Table 3.2). That would be approximately $2 \times 8$, or 16, when left and right halves of the body are considered. These would be Deep Radial-I (1); Great Auricular (2); Spinal Accessory-I (3); Saphenous-I (4); Deep Peroneal (5); Tibial-I (6); Greater Occipital (7); and Infraspinatus (8) (refer to Chapter 4). The reader should note that all of these,

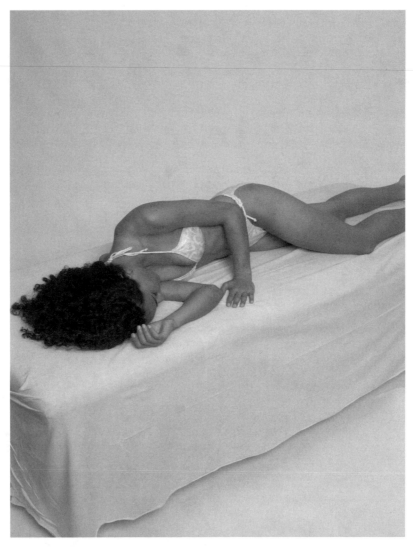

**FIGURE 8.3** The side position for acupuncture (note the leg position). The patient's center of gravity should be toward the anterior side of her body.

including the Greater Occipital but excluding the Infraspinatus and Deep Peroneal could be reached with the patient in a supine or a prone position.

Depending on the patient's problem, there will be some additional regional points in the passive or active phase. If the patient is having pain in the ankle, for example, the two Achilles (54), Inferolateral Malleolus (56), and Inferomedial Malleolus (57) points around the affected ankle might be tender, along with some unnamed nonspecific points. These might be more easily accessed with the patient in the supine position. Positioning in this case may not be too important: because many primary points are accessible whether the patient is prone or supine, the only real consideration is access to the tender local points around the area of injury. Alternating positions between the two usually makes the most sense. In this patient with a pain sensitivity of 1, only 20 points (16

tender primary points, 4 tertiary points, and a few nonspecific points) would be candidates for needling.

Compare a secondary patient. This person may have from 50 to 104 passive acupoints, plus the four tertiary points around the ankle and possibly a few other local nonspecific points. Whatever the patient's position, the tender points around the injured ankle, the accessible primary points, and some additional secondary points would be needled. Generally, a limit of 25 to 50 points needled in a session is appropriate for most patients. In any session, all the accessible primary points and the points around the ankle would be needled; then a reasonable number of secondary points would be added. The secondary points to be selected would be those along the nerve trunks leading to the affected ankle and then other accessible points, preferably those nearest the beginning of the sequence (those with the lowest numbers). The bottom line is that this higher degree patient will require more needles.

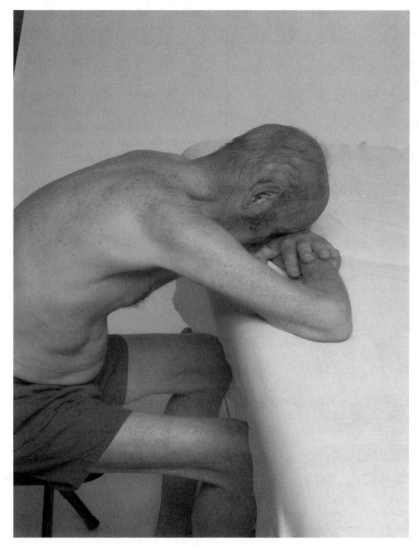

**FIGURE 8.4** The sitting position with the head resting on an examining table to avoid syncope. This position allows for needles to be placed on anterior and posterior surfaces of the body in the same session.

It becomes routine to needle the primary points because this is done in virtually every session. When needling only the primary points using the prone position, the following choices of points to needle seem reasonable:

- Greater Occipital (7)
- Spinal Accessory-I (3)
- Infraspinatus (8)
- Dorsal Scapular (13)
- Spinous Process of T7 (20)
- Posterior Cutaneous of T6 (21)
- Superior Cluneal (14)
- Posterior Cutaneous of L5 (22)
- Posterior Cutaneous of L2 (15)
- Inferior Gluteal (16)
- Iliotibial-I (18)
- Lateral Popliteal (11)
- Sural-I (10)

When the patient is supine, the following points would be appropriate:

- Great Auricular (2)
- Lateral Pectoral (17)
- Lateral Antebrachial Cutaneous (9)
- Deep Radial-I (1)
- Superficial Radial-I (12)
- Iliotibial-I (18)
- Saphenous-I (4)
- Common Peroneal-I (24)
- Tibial-I (6)
- Deep Peroneal (5)

Of course, this is not the only combination that could be used, but it is helpful for the practitioner to have a set routine for the primary points because they are used in almost every session. The sequences given would allow

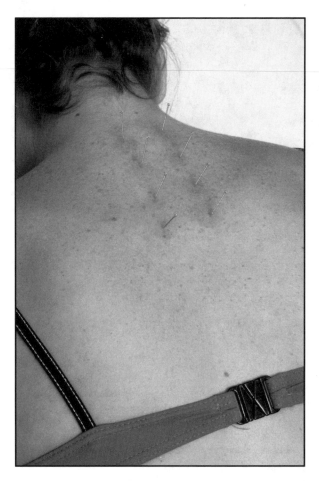

**FIGURE 8.5** The paravertebral points. Note the histamine reaction around the needles. Any physiological reaction to needling, such as this histamine reaction or sweating, is a sign that the patient is more likely than not to respond to acupuncture.

for 26 primary points to be needled when the patient is prone and 20 when the patient is supine. The points are listed more or less in the order in which they would be needled, moving from head to toe, with the exception that, in the low back, it is often convenient for the practitioner to start furthest away from him and work towards himself, to avoid having to work around needles already placed. Similarly, it is common to place all the needles practicable standing on one side of the patient's body and then to change sides (this would change the sequences cited somewhat). The sequence of placement is mostly a matter of convenience for the practitioner.

It is good practice occasionally to needle the area of the sympathetic trunk in the upper thoracic region by placing needles about 3 cm to each side of each spinous process from T2 to T6 (exact placement is not critical). These acupoints are collectively called Paravertebral points and are depicted in Figure 8.5. It is felt that this stimulates the sympathetic nervous system, possibly exhausting some neurotransmitters and generally reducing the patient's stress level. The only evidence supporting this practice is empirical and it should be noted that patients most commonly report being more relaxed and sleeping better after acupuncture, regardless of whether the Paravertebral points are needled. Nonetheless, the authors of this text routinely include these points some of the time when their patients are in the prone position. These points have special applicability to the conditions of allergy and asthma, as will be discussed in subsequent chapters.

In Chapter 11, a case will be described in detail as an example of applying principles discussed in this chapter to treatment of migraine headaches. The next two chapters discuss complications to be anticipated, equipment, and insertion technique. The complications are usually trivial and rarely dramatic. Obtaining and maintaining high-quality needles is an important consideration. Insertion technique is simple with several variations, depending on the preferences of the clinician. After these two chapters, the focus shifts to the treatment of specific conditions.

# 9 Complications of Treatment and Other Physiological Reactions

## CONTENTS

## 9.1 MAJOR COMPLICATIONS

Major complications are rare and include pneumothorax, pericardial tamponade, infection, and syncope. Deaths have been associated with acupuncture: in one case, an 82-year-old woman used a sewing needle to treat her angina and punctured her anterior interventricular artery;[1] two other patients died of staphylococcal septicemia.[2] Pneumothorax is frequently reported, but fortunately most cases produce only small collapses.[3–5] Hepatitis infection is the most commonly reported serious complication, but this is entirely avoidable.[6–9] Other serious complications involve failure to treat an underlying, life-threatening condition such as appendicitis, abdominal distention, peritonitis, acute cholecystitis, and cerebral malaria.[10] Other major complications include damage to ear cartilage with *auriculopuncture* (acupuncture of the external ear)[11,12] and damage to the spinal cord and associated structures.[13,14]

By far the most commonly experienced serious complication is syncope, especially when patients are needled in the sitting position. If the patient falls as a result, broken bones and head injuries can occur. Syncope may be preceded by coughing; sneezing; micturition; vomiting; and profuse diaphoresis. When these signs develop or the patient complains of light-headedness, it is advisable to remove all needles quickly and to move the patient to a head-down position, or if this is not practical, to a recumbent position with the head turned to the side to facilitate clearing the airway if he or she should vomit. (Diaphoresis alone when the patient is recumbent may not require the abrupt ending of a session; it is not uncommon for a prone patient, for example, to develop a pool of perspiration in the small of his or her back as a physiological reaction to needling. At a minimum, however, in this setting, the patient should be queried about nausea and light-headedness, and if the answers suggest a more serious reaction, the session should probably be ended.)

A needle placed in the skin of the face at the Depressor Septi (94) acupoint (or, if a needle is not available, forceful direct pressure with a fingernail) will usually revive the patient immediately. Another effective technique is to prick one of the patient's index fingertips with a needle. If syncope is not treated quickly, it may progress to a rare state in which the patient becomes as rigid as if in rigor mortis. This is frightening for the clinician but easily managed as described earlier; the response to removing the needles and inserting one in the depressor septi is immediate and dramatic. If the patient is still desirous of receiving acupuncture treatments after a major syncopal event, the practitioner may wish to start the next session with just a few needles and slowly increase the number from session to session until it is clear that syncope will not recur. One might wish to avoid using the sitting position to minimize the risk of syncope in a susceptible patient. Generally, use of the head-down sitting position depicted in Figure 8.4 is designed to minimize the possibility of a syncopal event.

This book is intended for physicians, and it is to be remembered that many acupuncturists in the world have no medical training. The experienced physician will readily recognize that, with the exception of syncope, these complications are avoidable. First and foremost, acupuncture should be used only when an established diagnosis has been established as well as an appropriate plan of treatment initiated for the underlying condition. The primary use of acupuncture is in managing pain; it cannot cure appendicitis or any of the other serious conditions described previously. It cannot be emphasized enough that acupuncture is for symptomatic relief of a

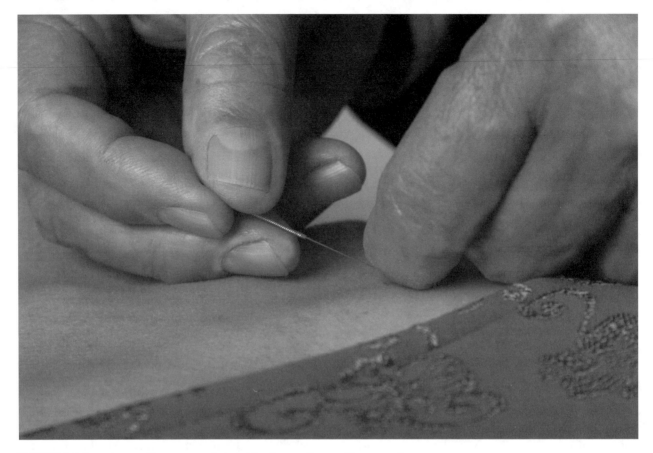

**FIGURE 9.1** Inserting needles at an angle in a thin chest wall to avoid pneumothorax.

well-understood underlying condition. Hopefully, no physician would attempt to treat an acute abdomen or crushing chest pain with needles.

Many other complications can be prevented by avoiding high-risk areas of the body unless the practitioner has a complete understanding of the underlying anatomy; the chest wall and the anterior neck are the only areas recommended for acupuncture in this text that have a significant risk of sustaining injury. Pneumothorax can be avoided by inserting needles superficially so that the pleura is not punctured; in exceptionally thin individuals, the needles may need to be inserted at an angle as shown in Figure 9.1. The anterior neck contains several structures, primarily vascular, that should be avoided; needles do not need to be inserted into the anterior neck except in rare cases (difficult cases of allergy and asthma, and chronic cough), so this is seldom a problem.

Although the literature cited earlier includes cases of infection and other injury to the spinal cord, it is unlikely that the careful reader of this text would ever insert a needle into the central nervous system. Superficial needles may be placed over spinous processes; these are most unlikely to enter the spinal canal. Needles placed a few centimeters to either side of the spine are similarly unlikely to be a problem to the spinal cord.

Infection such as hepatitis or HIV is a more serious concern: proper needle hygiene is an important topic covered in the next chapter.

## 9.2 MINOR COMPLICATIONS

It is inevitable that needles will produce bleeding from time to time. Bleeding will present as an ecchymosis or, occasionally, as a hematoma, or as a drop of blood on the skin after a needle is removed. This is more common in the elderly and, naturally, in those taking anticoagulants. It is rarely a problem but it is important to warn patients about the possibility before it happens to them. When needles are removed at the end of a session, the assistant should have a cotton ball or gauze pad available to blot up the inevitable few drops of blood from a few of the needles.

Patients often complain that a particular needle site, typically the Superficial Radial-I (12), hurts for some time after the needle is removed. Reassurance is all that is needed for this problem. Some may complain that a number of sites continue to experience pain or itching (as a result of a histamine reaction at the needle site) for some time after the needles are removed. Still others will complain of an increase in the pain for which they are getting treatment, especially after the first treatment session in their lives or after a long treatment hiatus (more than a year). This temporary flare-up of pain is quite common, especially in low-degree individuals; although it is not serious, it is one of the most common causes of patients' abandoning treatment. It can be minimized by using fewer needles during that first session. Patients should definitely be warned about this possibility and, if appropriate, counseled to begin the first session at a time when a possible flare-up will not seriously inconvenience them. (A recent case involved a student with a sensitivity of zero suffering from neck and shoulder pain who wanted to alleviate the pain so she could study for her exam the next day; she ended up postponing the exam because of the flare-up that ensued.)

Drowsiness and sleeplessness are both common, the latter often associated with pain flare-ups. Drowsiness may be associated with endorphin release in the central nervous system. Often patients will relate that they had the best night's sleep in years after a first acupuncture session; unfortunately, this reaction is not consistent (some patients report hyperactivity) and does not persist long enough to be useful as a treatment for insomnia.

Parasympathetic enhancement, as manifested by better control of urinary incontinence, relief of constipation and bowel irregularity, and decrease in blood pressure, may occur. Most patients would hardly consider these to be complications; unfortunately, they are usually transient. Additionally, there are better treatments than acupuncture for incontinence and bowel problems. Good evidence was presented in Dung's earlier text[15] that another effect of this parasympathetic enhancement may be increased fertility; in that work he describes how 7 of 16 infertility patients, having tried all other available treatments, became pregnant and produced healthy infants after acupuncture. Again, whether this is a complication or a benefit depends on the patient's perspective; it seems prudent to warn fecund patients of this possibility, especially if one is practicing in a state in which the negligence laws recognize a cause of action for "wrongful life," that is, an unwanted childbirth. It would seem that gynecologists who treat infertility should try acupuncture before undertaking more expensive and emotion-laden work-ups and treatments.

## 9.3 IMMEDIATE REACTIONS

Syncope, the most serious immediate reaction, was discussed earlier as a major complication. During the acupuncture session, other less serious physiological reactions to needles are frequently observed. A histamine-mediated atopic erythroid skin reaction is often observed as a 1- to 2-cm zone of erythema around the needle site. This reaction was depicted in Figure 8.5 in the previous chapter. Diaphoresis may occur; if extreme, this may be a harbinger of syncope, but usually is of no consequence. The sweating is a "cold sweat," most likely mediated by epinephrine, possibly along with other neurotransmitters. It is most frequent in patients between 25 and 45 years of age and is more common in males than in females. Hormonal reactions during the treatment session are frequently encountered in females and present with unexplained sadness and crying; this is more common early in the course of treatment. All of these reactions should be seen as beneficial, predicting a good eventual response to acupuncture; however, the patient should be forewarned.

## REFERENCES

1. Schiff, A.F. A fatality due to acupuncture. *Med. Times* 93:630, 1965.
2. Pierik, M.G. Fatal staphylococcal septicemia following acupuncture: report of two cases. *R.I. Med. J.* 65:251, 1982.
3. Gray, R. et al. Pneumothorax resulting from acupuncture. *Can. Assoc. Radiol. J.* 42:139, 1991.
4. Wright, R.S. et al. Bilateral tension pneumothoraces after acupuncture. *West J. Med.* 154:102, 1991.
5. Goldberg, I. Pneumothorax associated with acupuncture. *Med. J. Aust.* 1:941, 1973.
6. Boxall, E.H. Acupuncture hepatitis in the West Midlands. *J. Med. Virol.* 2:377, 1978.
7. Stryker, W.S. et al. Outbreak of Hepatitis B associated with acupuncture. *J. Fam. Pract.* 22:155, 1986.
8. Kent, G.P. et al. A large outbreak of acupuncture-associated Hepatitis B. *Am. J. Epidemiol.* 127:591, 1988.
9. Slater, P.E. et al. An acupuncture-associated outbreak of Hepatitis B in Jerusalem. *Eur. J. Epidemiol.* 4:322, 1988.
10. Rich, N.M. and Dimond, F.C. Results of Vietnamese acupuncture seen at the Second Surgical Hospital. *Mil. Med.* 132:791, 1967.
11. Davis, O. et al. Auricular perichondritis secondary to acupuncture. *Arch. Otolaryngol.* 111:770, 1985.
12. Savage Jones, H. Auricular complications of acupuncture. *J. Laryngol. Otol.* 99:1143, 1985.
13. Hadden, W.A. et al. Spinal infection caused by acupuncture mimicking a prolapsed intervertebral disc. *J. Bone Joint Surg.* 64:624, 1982.
14. Kondo, A. et al. Injury to the spinal cord produced by acupuncture needles. *Surg. Neurol.* 11:155, 1979.
15. Dung, H.C. *Anatomical Acupuncture.* Antarctic Press, San Antonio, 1997.

# 10 Needles, Accessories, and the Treatment Session

## CONTENTS

## 10.1 ACUPUNCTURE NEEDLES

For purposes of this text, needle technique is of more concern than the use of other techniques often included within the scope of acupuncture practice: so-called laser acupuncture, electrical acupuncture, moxibustion, cupping, and other variations. In general, the authors avoid the use of these other techniques; some are dangerous, some are ineffective, some are a nuisance, and most are unnecessary affectations. The stimulation provided by needles is safe, consistent, and readily performed without the need of elaborate preparation; it is difficult to imagine that adjuncts offer any improvement on this basic and essential skill. These other techniques will be described in this chapter, however, despite the authors' generally poor opinion of most of them.

The needle consists of a sharp tip, body, handle, and tail, as illustrated in Figure 10.1. The tip is typically 9 to 11 μm thick — thinner tips are prone to breaking and thicker ones are relatively difficult to insert. The body and tip are almost always made of stainless steel, although silver and gold have been touted by some as more "powerful." The handle often contains silver as an alloy that turns dark after repeated autoclaving. The tail is used by some (not the authors) for fastening burning materials; the heat is transmitted down the needle for further stimulation and, quite possibly, nerve damage.

Needles are available in lengths (of needle bodies) from 0.5 to 6 in. or more. A good assortment to begin with would be 0.5-in., 32-gauge; 1-in., 32-gauge; and 1.5- or 2-in., 30-gauge needles. The smaller needles are used primarily in the face; the midsize ones in the upper extremities, upper back (e.g., from T7 upward) and front of the chest; and the longer ones in the low back and legs. An assortment of disposable needles is shown in Figure 10.2.

Acupuncture has been practiced for many centuries and thus the history of acupuncture needles reflects the technology of the times. Prior to 1955, most needles were made by hand. Typically, each acupuncturist made his own needles. Good needles were kept as long as possible, often until they broke off in the flesh of a patient. Mass-produced needles began to appear around 1955. The first were made in Taiwan or Hong Kong, but now almost all come from China. Even though they are mass produced, they are inconsistent in quality; the most common variation is in the length of the body. Older acupuncturists may straighten needles that bend, but that invariably weakens the metal. Acupuncturists beginning practice today would be best advised to obtain disposable needles from a reputable supplier* and discard them once they are bent or otherwise damaged.

Even though they are labeled for disposable use, modern needles may be cleaned in alcohol or other solutions intended for cleaning surgical instruments and then autoclaved. Autoclaving alone is sufficient. Some practices give patients the option of purchasing "disposable nee-

---

* The needles pictured in this chapter were purchased from C A I Industries, 800 S. Palm Ave., Ste. 10, Alhambra, California 91803, (800) 234-8583. The authors have no financial interest in this company.

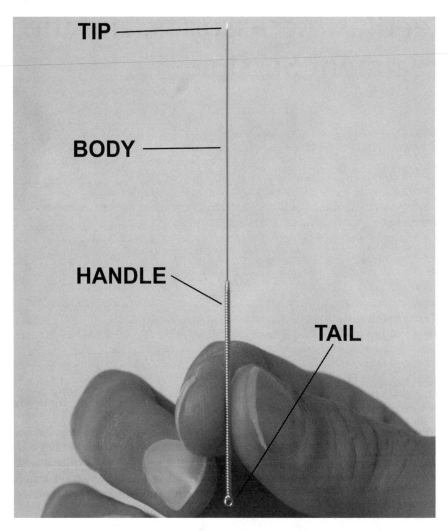

**FIGURE 10.1** An acupuncture needle, showing its sharp tip, slender body, somewhat thicker twisted handle, and open tail.

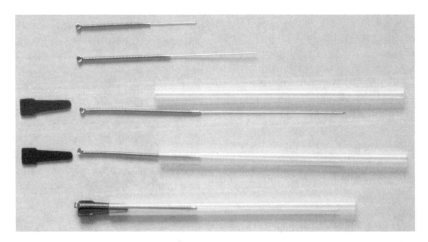

**FIGURE 10.2** Typical disposable needles and their inner packaging. Three lengths are shown (0.5, 1.0, and 2.0 in.). The bottom needle is in its inner packaging; the needle above it has the plastic stay removed and the middle needle has been removed from its plastic sheathing.

dles" if they are squeamish about sterilized needles; this simply means that unused needles are unpacked in front of the patient, used in the treatment session, and, once the session is complete, added to those to be sterilized for reuse. Dung has the most experience with reusing needles, having placed approximately 5 million needles in 16,000 patients during his 30-year career; neither he nor the other two authors have ever had a known case of infectious disease passed from one patient to another through reuse of needles. The authors feel justified in their conclusion, based on this history, that resterilization of needles is safe. However, it is imperative that trained personnel use strict procedures in resterilization because, undoubtedly, marginally trained personnel are responsible for the transmission of hepatitis C and other diseases through sloppy practices. If any doubt exists about the personnel and procedures involved, reuse of needles is to be discouraged.

Needles are reused, not because of the cost — a trivial 3 or 4 cents per needle — but because of the tedium of unwrapping new ones. They are packaged in boxes of 100 needles and each of the needles within the box is individually encased in a plastic sleeve with a small plastic stopper at one end (see Figure 10.2). These needles with their sleeves are packaged, again individually, in paper (on one side) and plastic (on the other). Five or so of these individually packaged needles are manufactured together in a strip separated by perforations. A hundred needles so packaged are packed in a box that is then wrapped in clear plastic. Once the box is unwrapped and opened, the needles can be unwrapped five at a time using the technique shown in Figure 10.3a through Figure 10.3h. Even so, this is a tedious and time-consuming task that is largely avoided by reusing the needles. Eventually, needles wear out or become dull and should be replaced. Long needles tend to bend on insertion and thus need to be discarded more often than shorter ones, especially when using the thinner gauges.

## 10.2 NEEDLE STORAGE AND STERILIZATION

Needles are best stored in stainless steel cups with lids as shown in Figure 10.4. The sizes shown are designed for 0.5-, 1-, and 1.5-in. needles. The lids have soft material that will not dull the needles stuffed into the insides; cloth tape will work, as will thin circles of balsa wood. Cotton balls should not be used because they tend to come up when a needle is removed from the lid, bringing all the other needles along with them. Whatever tip padding is used, it should be able to withstand autoclaving. The cups and lids are not currently available in the U.S.; the ones shown in the figure are from Taiwan. They are so convenient that it would be worth one's effort to have them made at a machine shop.

Dirty needles are stored, tip up, in the cups, which are deep enough to prevent the tips from protruding above their lips. When the cups are full of dirty needles, they and the lids, open ends up, are placed side by side in an autoclave and sterilized. Then the lids are placed on the cups; the cups and lids turned upside down (lids down); the cups gently removed from the lids; and the lids, with the needle points down and the handles exposed for easy access, placed on a tray ready for use. This obviates the need to handle the individual needles and is by far the safest means of processing them. The only caveat is that care should be taken to assure that the dirty needles, when placed in the bottom of a container, do not protrude above the container's lip; this can be facilitated if the person removing the needles with one hand will hold the container in the other and gently swirl it as dirty needles are added. This helps the needles work their way to the bottom immediately. Of course, a replacement container should always be available because overfilling should be avoided. Discarded needles (those not suitable for resterilization) must be disposed of in an approved "sharps container" and disposed of as would any other hazardous medical waste, or they may be sterilized first and then discarded.

The process of handling the needles in the containers is depicted in Figure 10.5 and Figure 10.6. If the practitioner does not have containers available, he or she must devise another method for handling the needles and may find that using new needles each session is the most expedient option. Stoppered test tubes with a little cotton stuffed tightly into the bottom can be used as containers, one set for clean ones and another for dirty ones; they are particularly convenient for traveling. The tubes for the dirty needles do not need to have cotton because the tips are placed pointing up toward the stoppers. The stoppers are carefully removed and the tubes and stoppers are placed into an autoclave for sterilizing.

## 10.3 ACUPUNCTURE ACCESSORIES AND ALTERNATIVES TO NEEDLES

*Moxibustion* has been mentioned previously. It is acupuncture associated with burning materials tied to the end of the acupuncture needles, waved over the body, or placed directly on the skin. On one hand, it is a metaphysically based purification ritual called "smudging" by its practitioners because the smoke is thought to cleanse the air of negative energies. On the other hand, it is an effort to add a component of heat to the surface of the body (by placing burning material as a cone directly on the skin) or beneath the skin (by fastening the burning material to the tail of a needle). Moxibustion has no therapeutic effect and is dangerous in that it may burn the skin or a major nerve beneath it. If a practitioner believes that the effect of acupuncture is placebo (the authors do not), he or she may find that this

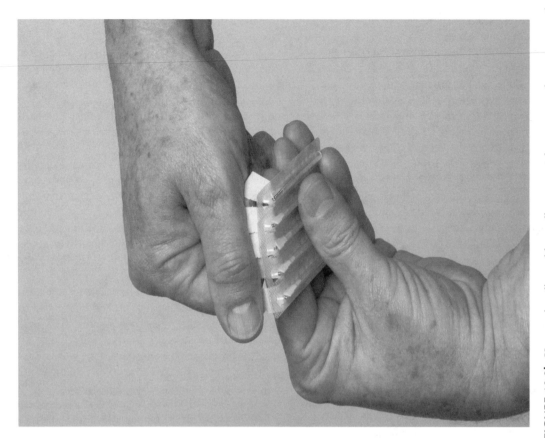

**FIGURE 10.3b** Unwrapping disposable needles: paper tabs are grasped as a group and pulled away from the plastic packaging.

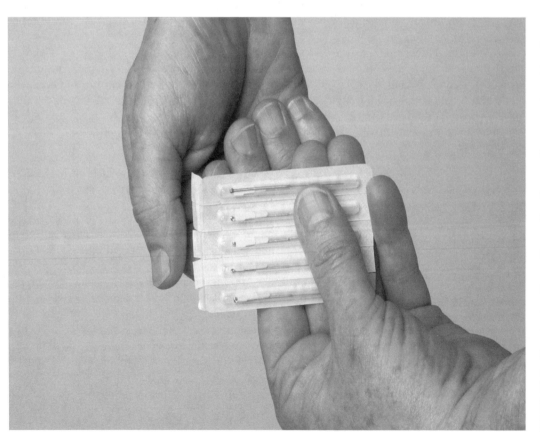

**FIGURE 10.3a** Unwrapping disposable needles: five needles are packaged together.

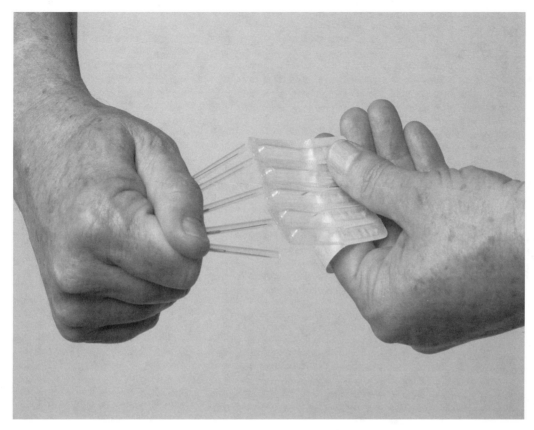

**FIGURE 10.3d** Unwrapping disposable needles: needles are grasped as a group and removed from the package.

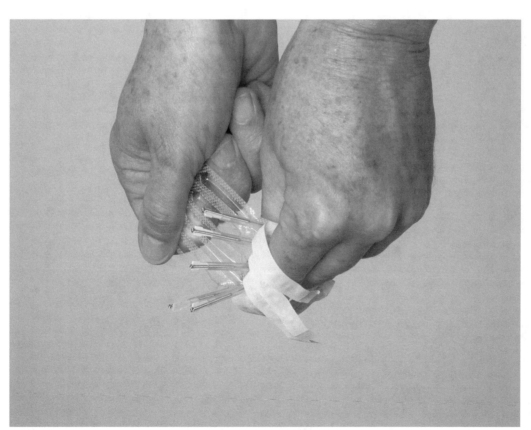

**FIGURE 10.3c** Unwrapping disposable needles: plastic packaging is bent back from the needles, exposing them.

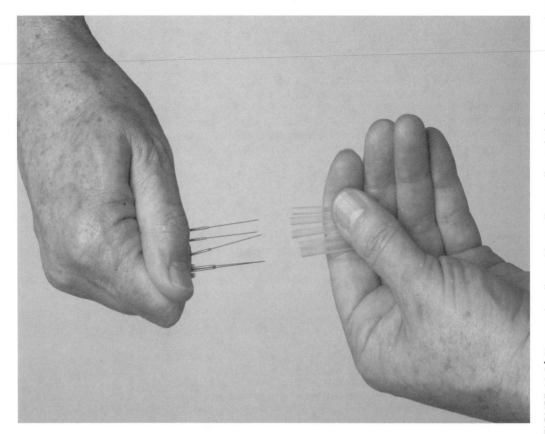

**FIGURE 10.3f** Unwrapping disposable needles: needles and plastic stays are removed as a group.

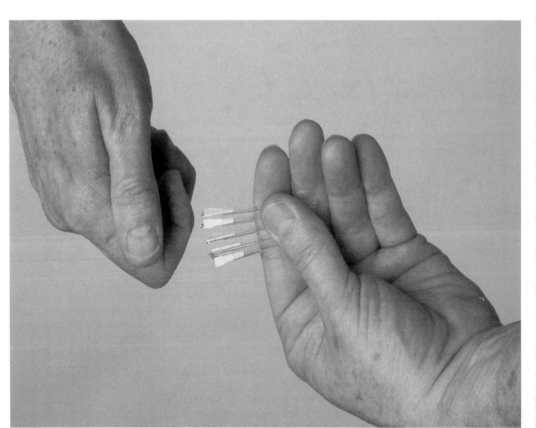

**FIGURE 10.3e** Unwrapping disposable needles: packaging is discarded and the needles in their sheaths are grasped by the free hand.

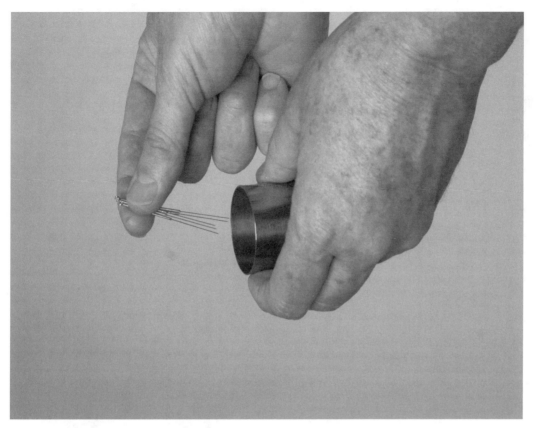

**FIGURE 10.3h** Unwrapping disposable needles: needles are stored in an appropriate container, in this case the lid of a stainless steel cup, with sterile padding in the bottom of the inverted lid to prevent dulling of the needle tips.

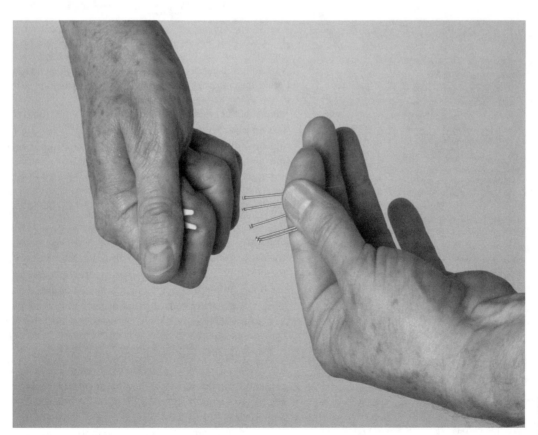

**FIGURE 10.3g** Unwrapping disposable needles: bodies of the needles are grasped by the free hand and stays are discarded.

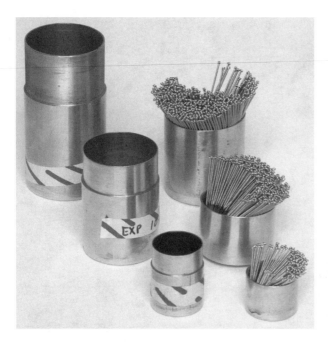

**FIGURE 10.4** Different sizes of cups can be used for different lengths of needles. Clean needles are stored in the lids and dirty needles are stored, tips up, in the bases.

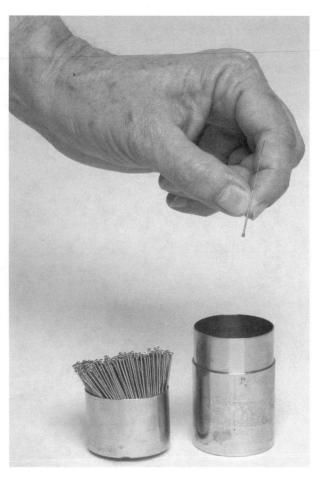

**FIGURE 10.6** A dirty needle is placed, tip up, in the base of the cup. The cup can be held in the nondominant hand and gently swirled as the needles are removed from the patient and dropped into it; this settles the needles so that no tips protrude above the rim.

bit of theater adds to the placebo effect. If not, moxibustion has no place in the physician's practice. It is time consuming and messy and converts a quick and simple practice into a circus.

*Cupping* is another affectation. It consists of placing a warmed open glass container (a juice glass would work) over the surface of the skin; as the gas within the container and the glass itself cool, a vacuum is created. It may be done over unpierced skin or over a needle; when the former is done, it is thought to drain negative energy from the body; with the latter, it is said to draw bad blood from the body. When it is placed over a needle inserted into the skin, it may create bleeding and occasionally a fairly large hematoma. Of course, if the glass is too hot, the patient can be burned.

*Acupressure* is a useful substitute for needles in very low-degree (primary) individuals. It consists of applying pressure to acupoints with the fingers or other devices (see Figure 10.7a and Figure 10.7b for a commercially available device). It can only be used in some areas of the body. It is painful for the practitioner to apply enough pressure

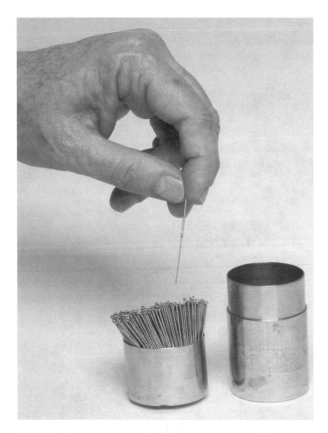

**FIGURE 10.5** A clean needle is selected from the lid of a cup.

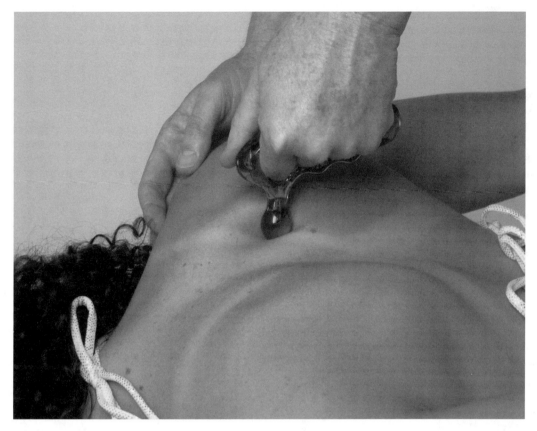

FIGURE 10.7b An acupressure device: in use on the medial border of the scapula.

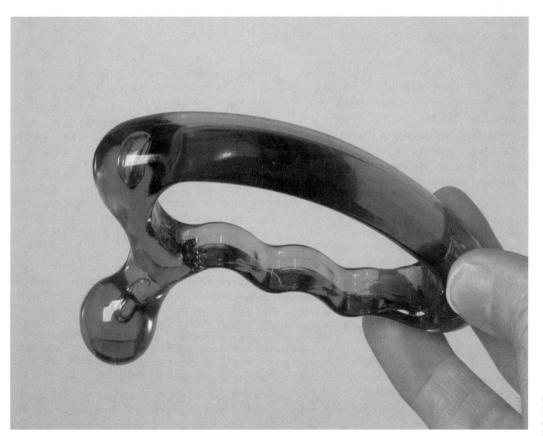

FIGURE 10.7a An acupressure device: close-up view.

with the hands to be effective, especially if it is done very frequently. The neck, shoulders, and back are amenable to this technique; however, sites over bony areas, e.g., Supraorbital (23), should not be used because the device used to apply pressure may slip and damage tissue, in this example the eye. This technique has two main drawbacks: it is blunt and capable of damaging a zone of tissue around the acupoint, and it is not possible to stimulate more than one or two acupoints at a time. Despite all the limitations, acupressure may be a useful expedient in low-degree individuals, especially when time is limited; furthermore, because it is noninvasive, it may be used by physical therapists and others under appropriate circumstances.

*Laser acupuncture* is inferior to needle acupuncture. It consists of stimulating acupoints with a low-intensity laser beam. Because the beam is of low power, it does not penetrate the skin but merely creates heat on the surface and immediately beneath it. Thus, it lacks the efficacy of needle stimulation of the nerve. Furthermore, it should be used with extreme caution around the eye because of the danger of producing retinal damage. The reader may note that some of the studies cited in Chapter 1 used laser acupuncture because it is easier to design a nontherapeutic look-alike for blinded use in controls than a needle. The problem with this approach is that the laser is less effective and the study is less likely to produce a statistically significant result. Again, it would be expected that laser acupuncture would only be effective in low-degree individuals.

*Electrical acupuncture* is, in the authors' estimation, a rather clumsy affectation that adds electrical stimulation to a needle. One device has six pairs of wires; each wire is connected to the tail of a needle and an alternating current is applied. There is no evidence that this does or does not increase the efficacy of acupuncture. The downside of this technique (other than expense of the equipment) is that it requires a nest of wires draped over the patient and precariously attached to the needles. Needles can be pulled out inadvertently, possibly with some bleeding, and an unattended patient may find that distressing.

## 10.4 EAR STAPLES

Ear staples, also called press pins, are tiny needles used in auriculopuncture (see Figure 10.8). They are packaged with a clear adhesive backing that is placed in the ear with the staple; both are left in place for a period of about 2 weeks. The use of these needles is described in the next chapter in conjunction with our discussion of conditions of the face and head.

## 10.5 NEEDLE INSERTION

Most nociceptors are situated in the dermis and epidermis. To avoid needle insertion pain, needles should be inserted

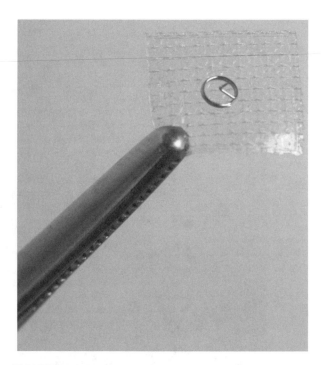

**FIGURE 10.8** Ear staple. The point is projecting toward the camera from the center of the staple.

in a manner so as to pierce these layers quickly and avoid pain during the insertion process. The plastic tubes packaged around commercially available disposable needles such as that shown in Figure 10.2 are designed to facilitate that purpose. Once the plastic stopper at the tail end of the needle is removed, the entire apparatus, needle and plastic tube, can be placed vertically on the skin surface as shown in Figure 10.9a. The tail of the needle, protruding above the tube several millimeters, can be tapped with a finger, causing the point to penetrate the skin surface quickly and reliably (Figure 10.9b). Then the sheath can be removed and discarded (Figure 10.9c) as the needle is advanced deeper. If a practitioner inserts needles rarely, this may be the best technique to use; note that it requires using new disposable needles. It is relatively slow, and anything that retards the process of needle insertion only increases a patient's discomfort. Nonetheless, it is safe and effective.

Far more elegant and efficient is to hold the needle in two hands as shown in Figure 10.10 and push the needle quickly with the upper hand (shown as the right hand in the figure) and guide it with the other, lower hand. The only problem with this method is a tendency of the needle body to bend instead of the tip penetrating; this is more of a problem with longer needles. A variation of this technique is to hold the needle as shown in Figure 10.11 but away from the skin, bringing both hands and the needle to, and through, the skin surface in one movement and then following through with the upper hand to insert the

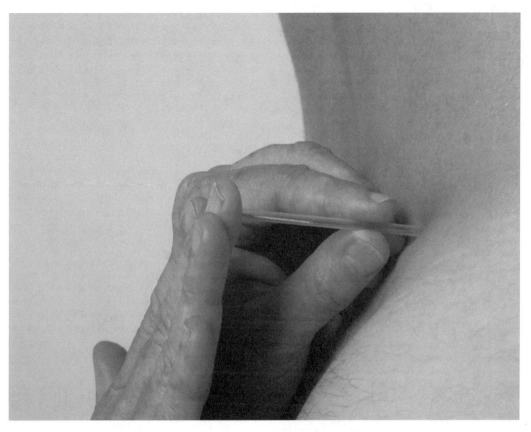

**FIGURE 10.9b** One method of insertion of a disposable needle packed in a plastic tube (continued): the tail of the needle is tapped firmly, driving the tip quickly into the skin.

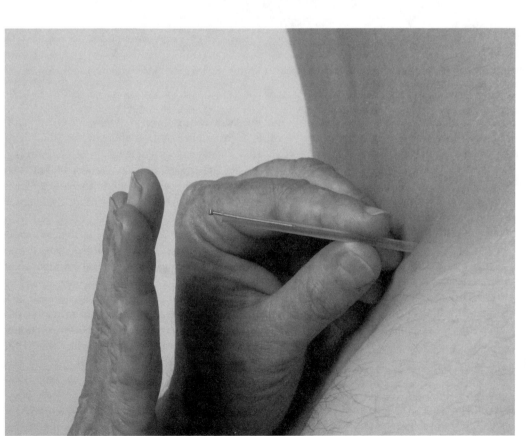

**FIGURE 10.9a** One method of insertion of a disposable needle packed in a plastic tube: the tip of the needle barely rests on the skin inside the sheath, protruding a few millimeters out of the tube as the practitioner's hand is poised to strike it.

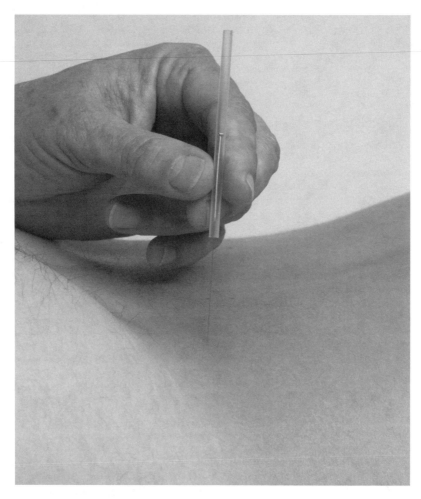

**FIGURE 10.9c** One method of insertion of a disposable needle packed in a plastic tube (continued): the sheath is removed and the needle is manually advanced to the desired depth.

needle to the required depth. This avoids the bending problem because the insertion force is applied with the lower hand. At any rate, this is a matter of experience and personal preference, and the beginning practitioner is encouraged to use his own exposed anterior thigh as an ideal target for practice.

When a large number of needles is inserted, it is preferable to learn to store additional needles between the index and middle fingers of the lower hand as depicted in Figure 10.10 and Figure 10.11. This requires quite a bit of practice but can be learned eventually. This is an important skill to make the insertion process quicker and thus a less negative experience for the patient. Inserting 30 to 50 needles should take from 3 to 5 minutes.

## 10.6 STERILE TECHNIQUE

It may be discomfiting for some practitioners to accept the fact that sterile technique is not strictly followed when performing acupuncture. It is virtually impossible to han-

dle needles wearing surgical gloves, for one thing. It has been the experience of the authors that washing the hands with a disinfectant soap immediately before inserting needles is adequate. Furthermore, the skin is not routinely prepped prior to needle insertion. Theoretically, a small amount of bacteria from the skin surface could be carried beneath the skin by the tip and body of the needle, but in practice the authors have never experienced problems from not prepping. (Dung has placed approximately 5 million needles over a 30-year career without an infection.) Generally, complaints about itching around needle sites in the hours after acupuncture are a result of histamine reaction to the needles occurring at the time of insertion, rather than to infection or bodily reaction to the stainless steel of the needles. If the reader is unwilling to follow the authors' practice, he could have an assistant stand on the other side of the patient and prep sites with alcohol sponges immediately prior to insertion. Of course, it would not be advisable to insert needles through grossly contaminated skin without first cleansing it.

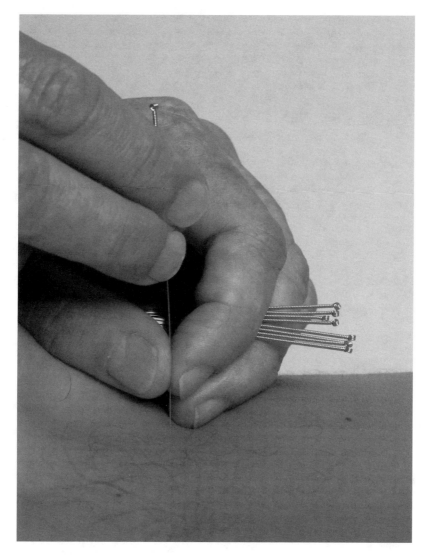

**FIGURE 10.10** Two-handed method of inserting needles without the use of a tube (see text).

## 10.7 ANGLE AND DEPTH OF INSERTION

Most acupuncture needles are inserted perpendicularly to the skin surface. The exception is those areas over the lungs when pneumothorax in an exceptionally thin patient is possible; in this instance, angled insertion reduces the chance of piercing the pleura (shown in Figure 9.1 in the previous chapter). Angled needles are also used to penetrate beneath the medial border of the scapula to access the Dorsal Scapular (13) point and to penetrate over the posterior iliac crest to access the Superior Cluneal (14) point. This latter important point may require an exceptionally long needle to access completely in an obese individual.

The depth of insertion depends on anatomical considerations. In the face, acupoints are often formed where the nerves come through bony foramina; needles should not be inserted into the foramina, but only into the skin superficial to the foramina. Thus, short needles are typically used. Because shorter needles are easily inserted, even with one hand, the other hand can be used to bunch up the skin to avoid penetrating the underlying structures accidentally (see Figure 10.12). The presence of the hand bunching up the skin also protects structures, e.g., eyes, to the sides of the acupoint. In the upper thorax and upper extremities, 1-in. needles are suitable. In the low back and lower extremities, longer needles, 1.5 to 2.0 in., are used, and some practitioners may use even longer needles for the Superior Cluneal (14) points in obese individuals. When spare needles are held as shown in Figure 10.10, they should not be held over the eyes because they may be inadvertently dropped.

There is a practical consideration in choosing needle length. The same size needles should be used consistently throughout a body region and this consistency should be maintained, as much as possible, from patient to patient.

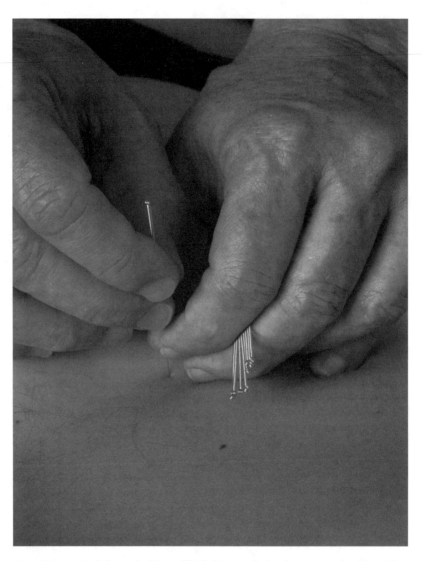

**FIGURE 10.11** A variation of the method shown in Figure 10.10. The needle is advanced to the skin with the tip slightly protruding and held firmly by the lower hand; once the skin is penetrated, the grip of the lower hand is loosened and the upper hand advances the needle deeper.

Following such a practice makes it more likely that the needles will be properly sorted by length as they are removed by an assistant.

## 10.8 COURSE OF A TREATMENT SESSION

It is good practice, even in a familiar patient who has had many acupuncture sessions, to greet the patient before the patient is disrobed and positioned. After the patient is disrobed to the extent necessary and positioned and draped by an assistant (preferably of the same gender as the patient), the practitioner enters the room, washes his hands, and begins placing the needles. The assistant remains in the room and observes where the needles are placed; this prevents the assistant from failing to remove needles that are partially obscured (particularly by hair) or placed in unusual locations. It is good practice to point

out needles in obscure locations to the assistant while the needles are being inserted.

A timer is started for 7 minutes; if the patient has not experienced acupuncture before or otherwise requests not to be left unattended, the assistant can sit with the patient while waiting for the timer alarm to sound. When left alone, patients should be asked whether they want the room lights left on, off, or (if possible) dimmed. It is also good practice always to leave an attendant with a new patient, particularly a female who may experience a sudden onset of sadness and crying as described in the preceding chapter. Patients receiving acupuncture in the sitting position should not be left alone because of the possibility of syncope. Generally, though, experienced patients are unconcerned about being left alone for a few minutes.

Once the timer sounds, the assistant "spins" or stimulates the needles (Figure 10.13). This is a time-honored

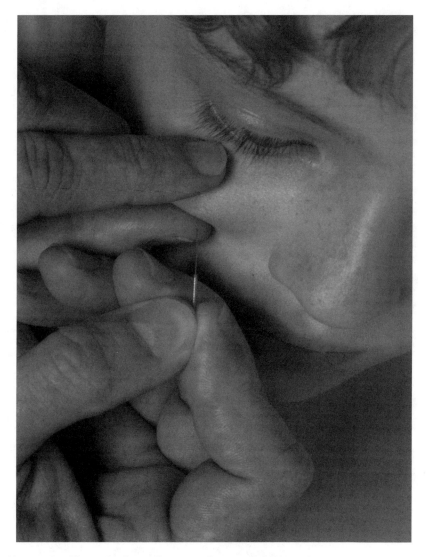

**FIGURE 10.12** Bunching up the skin on the face to insert needles superficially

practice that may or may not be necessary. *Spinning* consists of grasping the tail and handle of the needle and turning it slightly back and forth *once* between the thumb and index fingers to provide additional stimulation. Patients complain about exceedingly aggressive spinners. The timer is reset for another 7 minutes and, when it sounds, the needles are removed, the patient is left to get dressed, and a subsequent session is scheduled. The whole process takes from 20 to 25 minutes, and only about 5 minutes of the practitioner's time. One busy acupuncture practitioner will require at least three and preferably four or five treatment rooms.

Patients typically experience more intense pain in several (typically one to four) needle sites during the acupuncture session. This is normal. Sometimes they may complain loudly about one individual site. When this happens, it is often sufficient to manipulate the needle slightly, by spinning it or adjusting its depth. Sometimes it makes more sense simply to remove an offending needle entirely;

one is loathe to do this in an active site because the offending needle may be the one doing the most good. The practitioner and assistants should be careful when moving about the patient not to inadvertently brush against the ends of protruding needles, causing unwarranted additional stimulation.

## 10.9 THE NEW PATIENT AND FREQUENTLY ASKED QUESTIONS

Depending on the type of practice, new patients may present solely for the purpose of having acupuncture, or a physician may suggest it to a patient he or she is treating as a primary care physician or specialist. If the patient has not considered receiving acupuncture treatment prior to coming to the clinic, he or she may be very reluctant to receive needles, so the subject needs to be broached gingerly. One successful approach is to offer acupuncture to a patient only as an option, giving the patient some printed

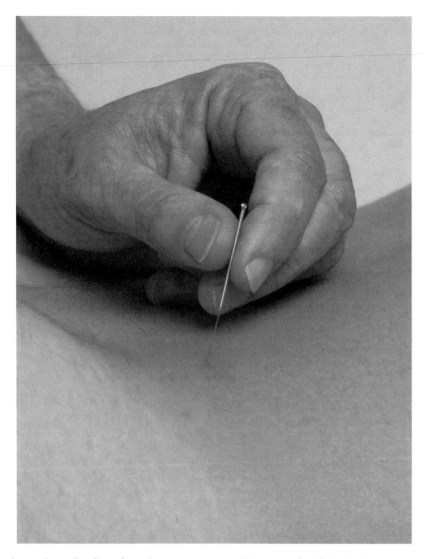

**FIGURE 10.13** Spinning each needle after a few minutes creates a small amount of additional stimulation, which may increase the efficacy of the entire procedure.

information and deferring the topic until the next appointment. Then, at the next appointment, the patient can be asked if he or she has decided to try acupuncture and his or her questions can be answered at this time.

Some patients, on the other hand, readily welcome an alternative to medication (although we are always careful to say that acupuncture is an alternative to medicine, but it is *not* "alternative medicine" — at least not the way we practice it). Patients will invariably ask if it hurts to have acupuncture; we invariably respond affirmatively, but add that the pain will be different from that which they are expecting. Patients expect pain like that often experienced from an injection; we tell them it is more of an aching pain than a sharp pain. It is sometimes helpful to show them that the needles are so small that they can be threaded into the bore of a small hypodermic needle. They will often have questions about

sterility and side effects. Regarding sterility, we typically explain that the needles are autoclaved, that we have never had an infection spread by needles, and that disposable needles are available for an extra charge. Regarding side effects, we explain that a patient may have an ugly bruise, that he or she will bleed a drop or two occasionally, and that pneumothorax is a remote possibility (although not in our experience).

These questions are also addressed in our "frequently asked questions" handout, along with advice to wear loose shorts and, for women, a tank top to the clinic when receiving acupuncture. Patients are also advised not to take pain medications before undergoing acupuncture. Women patients are also asked if they are pregnant because we consider this a contraindication to acupuncture treatment. It is advisable to have the patient sign an informed consent form.

# 11 Conditions of the Face and Head

## CONTENTS

## 11.1 INTRODUCTION TO SPECIFIC CONDITIONS BY ANATOMICAL REGION

This chapter begins an investigation of the uses of acupuncture in specific conditions; this and the following chapters are arranged by anatomical region. Of course, many conditions affect more than one region of the body and the lines of demarcation between regions are somewhat indistinct. Conditions have been grouped by the anatomical region most affected and those regions have been delineated primarily by their innervation. Also, a number of case histories are presented in this chapter, to illustrate not only specific conditions of the face and head but also the general principles of management discussed in the last few chapters.

## 11.2 OVERVIEW OF CONDITIONS OF THE FACE AND HEAD

This chapter primarily covers conditions of the face and head associated with the cranial nerves. Of the cranial nerves, the trigeminal (V) is the most important, followed by the spinal accessory (XI) and arguably the facial (VII), and finally by the glossopharyngeal (IX) and vagus (X). The facial (VII) is problematic because it is undetermined whether it contains afferent fibers for general sensation. Treatment of head and face pain with acupuncture generally involves these five cranial nerves, as does treatment of sinus allergy and asthma. Pain, primarily headache, is the most important application of acupuncture in the face and head. The back of the head is innervated primarily by cervical spinal nerves and is addressed in the next chapter's discussion of the neck and shoulders; however, the points in the back of the head and neck can be useful in addressing the conditions of the face and head discussed in this chapter.

Another important application of acupuncture in the face and head is the treatment of sinus allergy and asthma; this is gratifyingly successful in approximately 75% of patients *regardless of pain sensitivity level*. One author of this text found that the treatment of asthma in this way had an unexpected but significant benefit of controlling one patient's motion sickness as well. Sinus allergy is discussed later in this chapter.

Finally, the ear is the target of tiny needles, called staples or press pins, for the treatment of addictions such as smoking and overeating. These treatments can be made more effective with the addition of other modalities: visual imagery or hypnosis, group and individual counseling, and support groups. Medication may be a useful adjunct as well. Some of these addictions are discussed later in this chapter.

Conditions of the special senses are not very amenable to acupuncture. The olfactory (I), optic (II), and vestibulocochlear (VIII) nerves, for example, supply some of these senses, and no single acupoint is associated with or located along these three cranial nerves. Thus, acupuncture is not very useful for problems in which the primary pathology involves a deficit in a special sense organ, such as a loss in smell, vision, hearing, or equilibrium. Good examples of special sensory deficits associated with primary pathology in these cranial nerves are neurogenic deafness, retinitis pigmentosa, blindness resulting from destruction along the optic nerve, and loss of the sense of smell due to olfactory nerve transection (which occurs in a fracture of the cribriform plate of the ethmoid bone).

However, if the affected cranial nerve is intact without identifiable pathology and neuropathways connecting the cranial nerve to the central nervous system have no lesions, acupuncture may be successful in making modest improvements in some forms of hearing loss, smelling deficiency, and vision defect. Examples of special sense problems that acupuncture may help include certain forms of medication-induced tinnitus, loss of smelling sense due to chronic congestion of the nasal cavities, and blurred vision as a result of a mild increase in intraocular pressure. The basic approach to these conditions is not much different from the approach in treating headache: primary points throughout the body are treated while special attention is given to those of the head and face — particularly those around the affected organ. Of course, in all these conditions an accurate diagnosis and medical or surgical treatment of any underlying condition should take precedence over acupuncture treatments; the main advantage of physician-performed acupuncture is that attention is given to the entire patient and a broad range of possible causes and treatments is considered.

Before considering treatment of specific conditions, the practitioner should be aware of the neuroanatomy of the region, a brief review of which follows.

## 11.3 ACUPUNCTURE AND NEUROANATOMY OF THE HEAD AND NECK

As stated earlier, the trigeminal (V) is by far the most important cranial nerve to consider in the face and head, followed by the spinal accessory (XI), arguably the facial (VII), and occasionally the glossopharyngeal (IX) and vagus (X) nerves. Treatment of head and face pain with acupuncture generally involves these nerves, so it is beneficial to explore the neuroanatomy of each of them.

### 11.3.1 ACUPOINTS OF THE TRIGEMINAL NERVE (V)

Before emerging from the cranium, the trigeminal nerve divides into three divisions: ophthalmic (also known as V1), maxillary (V2), and mandibular (V3). The afferent fibers of this nerve converge at the semilunar, or trigeminal, ganglion. The mandibular division also contains efferent fibers from the motor nucleus of the trigeminal; this nucleus is buried inside the midbrain.

The ophthalmic division has many branches, but only four are relevant to this discussion: the supraorbital, supratrochlear, infratrochlear, and lacrimal. These are cutaneous nerves with eight acupoints along their distribution: the Supraorbital (23); Coronal Suture (71); Pterion (72); Bregma (75); Nasion (97); Frontalis (100); Lacrimal (102); and Supratrochlear (U). The derivation of the Frontalis is controversial, with some authorities attributing the efferent fibers to the facial nerve and the afferent fibers to the trigeminal. These points are depicted in Figure 11.1a and Figure 11.1b. The cutaneous nerves from this division innervate the area superior to the eyes to the top of the scalp. Each of these acupoints is discussed in more detail in the following paragraphs.

The Supraorbital (23) acupoint is formed at the site where the supraorbital nerve emerges through the supraorbital foramen. This foramen is the second largest of the face and the supraorbital nerve is the second largest nerve in the face. Not surprisingly, the acupoint at the emergence of the nerve through the foramen is the second facial acupoint to become tender in the progression of pain, after the Infraorbital (19). To locate the Supraorbital, visualize the eyebrow as divided into thirds; this point is located between the medial and middle thirds, on the superior margin of the eyebrow. The supraorbital artery and vein accompany the nerve at this point. The autonomic fibers mixed within the supraorbital nerve arise from the superior cervical ganglion of the sympathetic nervous system. It is important to note that it is neither necessary nor desirable for an acupuncture needle to enter the foramen; the skin

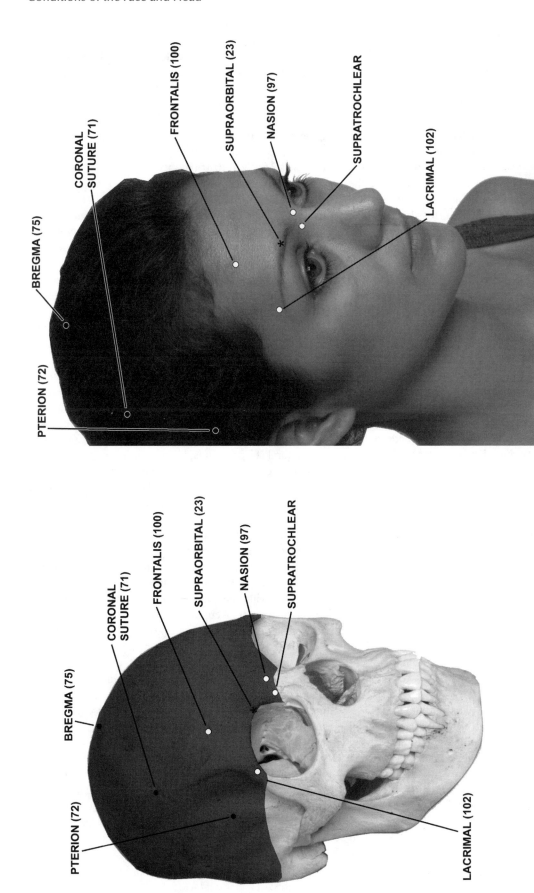

**FIGURE 11.1a** Acupoints of the face and head originating from the ophthalmic division (V1) of the trigeminal nerve: acupoints indicated on a human skull.

**FIGURE 11.1b** Acupoints of the face and head originating from the ophthalmic division (V1) of the trigeminal nerve: acupoints indicated on a live model.

area superficial to the foramen is richly innervated with fibers from the nerve beneath and stimulating those fibers is sufficient. An attempt to wedge a needle into the foramen would probably be unsuccessful and could easily damage the nerve and accompanying vessels.

The Lacrimal (102) acupoint is associated with small terminal branches of the lacrimal nerve that innervates the lacrimal gland, located behind the superolateral margin of the orbit. Tiny twig branches of the nerve run under the skin of the lateral one-third of the eyebrow, forming the lacrimal acupoint. Needles inserted into this point may be helpful in treating dryness and itching of the eye. The Bregma (75) acupoint is located where the coronal and sagittal suture lines of the skull join, at the site of the cartilaginous anterior fontanelle in infants. This fontanelle is the last to close, possibly accounting for the fact that skin over the bregma has richer innervation than the surrounding bony skull. The suture lines generally are likely to form acupoints, especially in patients with chronic headaches. The Coronal Suture (71) acupoint is another example of an acupoint along a suture line. The Pterion (72) acupoint is located at the site of the anterolateral fontanelle and receives its innervation from the supraorbital and the auriculotemporal nerves.

In discussing surface anatomy, the term *nasion* describes the midpoint between the medial ends of the two eyebrows. Skin of the nasion is innervated by small terminal branches of supraorbital and supratrochlear nerves. The Nasion (97) acupoint is very rarely used in acupuncture practice.

The Supratrochlear (U) and Infratrochlear (U) acupoints are formed by the supratrochlear and infratrochlear nerves, respectively. The nerves are very fine branches; the unnamed foramena through which they emerge are rarely visible in dry bony skulls dissected in gross anatomy classes. It seems that the foramena close as individuals age and the nerves disappear totally. Probably for this reason, the Supratrochlear and Infratrochlear points very rarely appear tender; an exception would be an individual with a longstanding problem, such as headaches present more than 20 years. The Supratrochlear is depicted in Figure 11.1a and Figure 11.1b.

The maxillary division (V2), like the ophthalmic division, consists of cutaneous nerves containing afferent and autonomic fibers emerging through foramena in the face. Fibers of this division are distributed to the area between the eyes and upper lip anterior to the ear, as well as to a portion of the ear. Acupoints are formed at the foramena through which these nerves emerge (see Figure 11.2a and Figure 11.2b).

V2 contains more parasympathetic nerve fibers than V1, a distinction that may explain how acupuncture works to relieve allergy symptoms. The parasympathetic fibers in V2 arise from neurons of the superior salivatory nucleus inside the brain between pons and medulla oblongata and

then join the facial nerve (VII) to go through the internal acoustic meatus. From there, these fibers depart from the facial nerve to enter a tiny groove — the greater petrosal sulcus. The fibers then go through the petrosal canal where they are called nerves of the petrosal canal and arrive at the pterygopalatine ganglion, from which postganglionic parasympathetic nerve fibers originate. The postganglionic parasympathetic fibers then divide and join the branches of V2 to distribute to the skin and epithelia of the head and face, including, importantly, the nasal cavities and the maxillary and sphenoid sinuses. The epithelia of the nasal cavities and sinuses are physiologically able to produce secretions controlled by the parasympathetic nerves. Because of the interconnection between the parasympathetic nerves and the nerves of V2, it is possible to modify secretory activities in the cavities and sinuses, and thus control sinus allergy, by stimulating acupoints on the face and nose. Four acupoints are formed by V2: the Infraorbital (19); the Zygomaticofacial (83); the Zygomaticotemporal (U); and the Paranasal (U).

Just below the inferior rim of the orbital fossa, the Infraorbital (19) acupoint is formed by the infraorbital nerve as it emerges through the infraorbital foramen, the largest of the face, to become cutaneous. This is the most important acupoint of the face and is essential in managing headache. The Zygomaticofacial (83) and the Zygomaticotemporal (U) acupoints, located at the emergence of the zygomaticofacial and zygomaticotemporal nerves through tiny foramena in the zygomatic bone, are relatively minor. If they are tender in a headache patient, the patient's prognosis is poor. The paranasal (U) acupoint, which is not a named anatomical landmark, is located at the junction of the wing of the nose and the face (Figure 11.2b and Figure 11.3). Few patients have tenderness at this point; however, it is a very useful point for symptoms associated with allergy, asthma, and other diseases of the respiratory tract. Acupuncture affects these symptoms through its effect on the rich postganglionic parasympathetic fibers in the area near the infraorbital nerve.

Unlike the other two divisions of the trigeminal nerve, the mandibular division (V3) includes efferent fibers that innervate the muscles of mastication. See Figure 11.4a and Figure 11.4b. Two neuromuscular attachments are formed by the branches of V3: the sites of the Masseter (30) and the Temporalis (59) acupoints. Six other acupoints in the distribution of V3 are cutaneous: the Mental (50); the triad of the Temporomandibular (27), Auriculotemporal (U), and Anterior Auricular (U); the Superior Auricular (51); and the Mentalis (U). The derivation of the Auriculotemporal and Anterior Auricular is assumed to be from V3, but this has not been completely determined because their anatomy is very complex. The mandibular division has two other unique characteristics: it carries (1) afferent fibers for the special sense of taste and (2) postganglionic parasympathetic

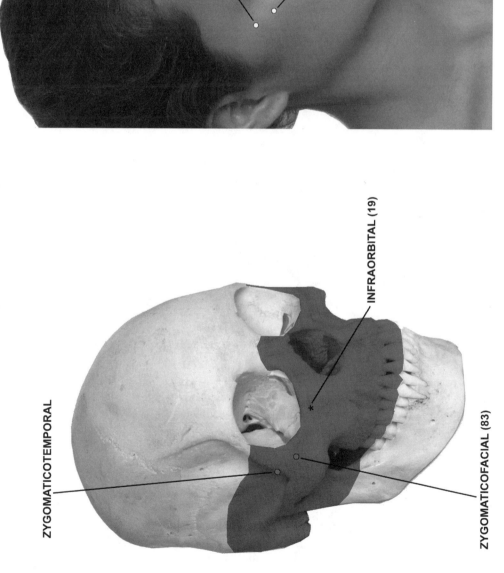

**FIGURE 11.2a** Acupoints of the face and head originating from the maxillary division (V2) of the trigeminal nerve: acupoints indicated on a human skull.

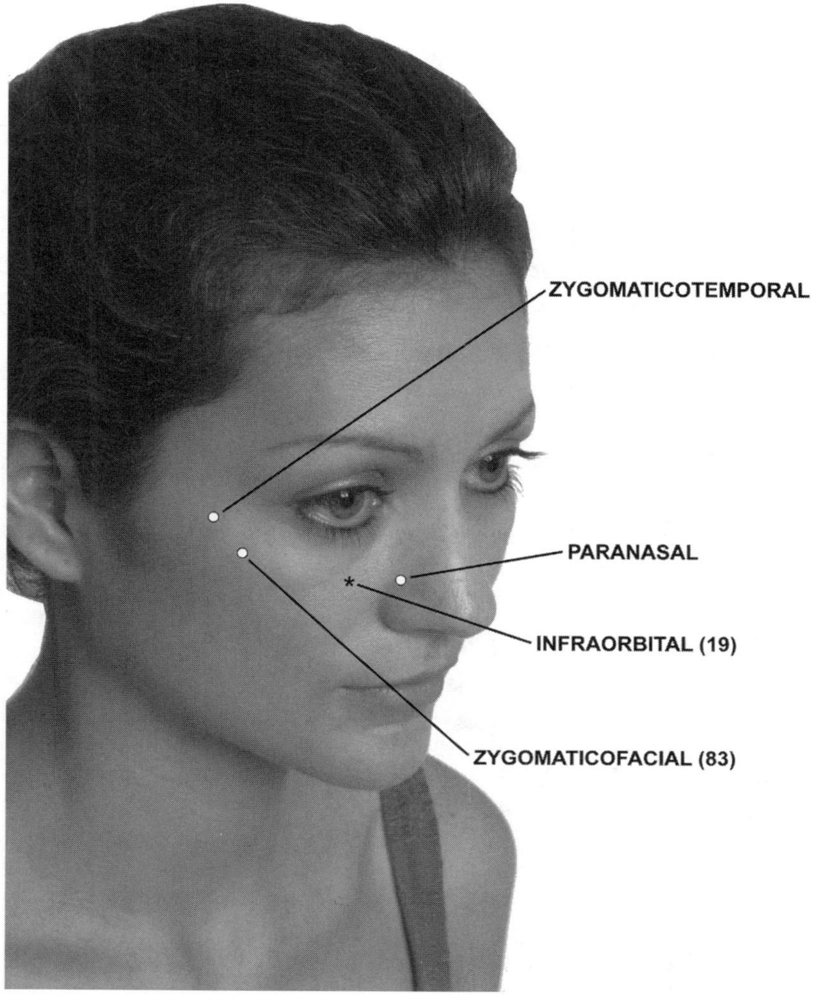

**FIGURE 11.2b** Acupoints of the face and head originating from the maxillary division (V2) of the trigeminal nerve: acupoints indicated on a live model.

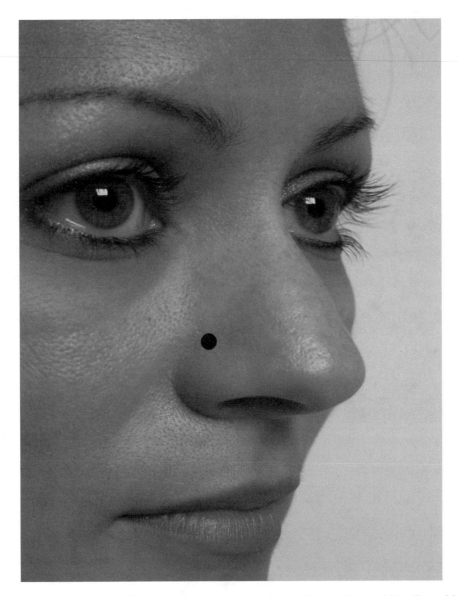

**FIGURE 11.3** The paranasal (U) acupoint (live model). A needle directed into this acupoint would be directed into the side of the nose (not into the cheek but parallel to it)

fibers to control secretion of glandular tissue in the oral cavity. Acupoints of V3 might be helpful in treating xerostomia, which is occasionally a complication of radiation therapy to the lower face. The reader should note that the afferent fibers for the special sense of taste travel from the tongue in the lingual nerve (V3) but at the chorda tympani diverge to join the facial nerve in its course to the brain.

The Mental (50) acupoint is located at the emergence of the mental nerve through the mental foramen in the mandible. This foramen is the third largest in the face and thus the Mental acupoint is not likely to become tender in the progression of chronic pain unless the nerves emerging from the two larger foramena have also become tender.

The Temporomandibular (27) acupoint is immediately superficial to the temporomandibular joint. This point is formed by innervation of the joint rather than by discrete nerve elements. Another point 1 cm superior to the Temporomandibular (27) and just anterior to the tragus of the ear is called the Auriculotemporal (U) acupoint. About 1 cm superior to this acupoint is the Anterior Auricular (U) acupoint. These three points are significant, particularly in patients with temporomandibular joint syndrome (TMJ) and headache, because they become tender in a predictable sequence with the progression of pain: first, the lower Temporomandibular (27) acupoint, followed by the Auriculotemporal (U) acupoint, and then by the Anterior Auricular (U) point. These points are secondary, tertiary, and nonspecific, respectively. See Figure 11.5, which also

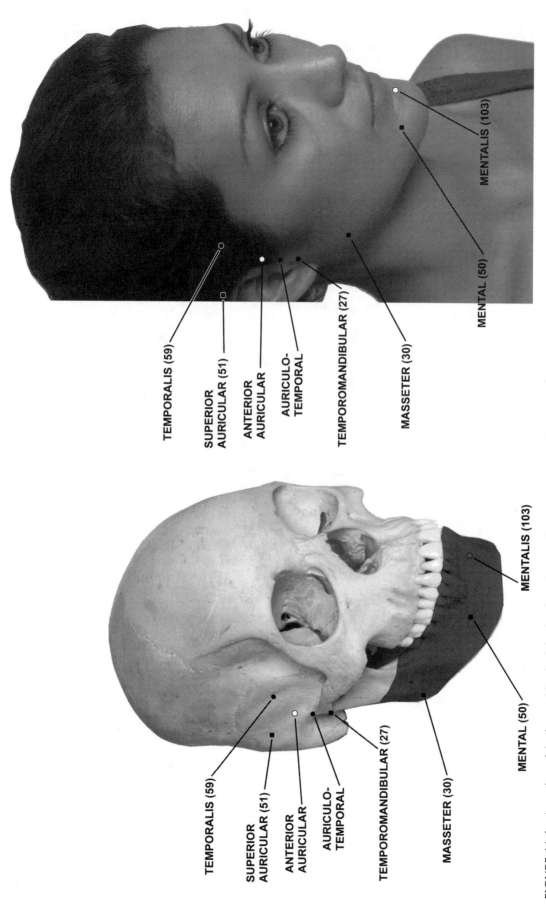

TEMPORALIS (59)

SUPERIOR AURICULAR (51)

ANTERIOR AURICULAR

AURICULO-TEMPORAL

TEMPOROMANDIBULAR (27)

MASSETER (30)

MENTAL (50)

MENTALIS (103)

**FIGURE 11.4b** Acupoints of the face and head originating from the mandibular division of the trigeminal nerve (live model).

**FIGURE 11.4a** Acupoints of the face and head originating from the mandibular division of the trigeminal nerve (human skull).

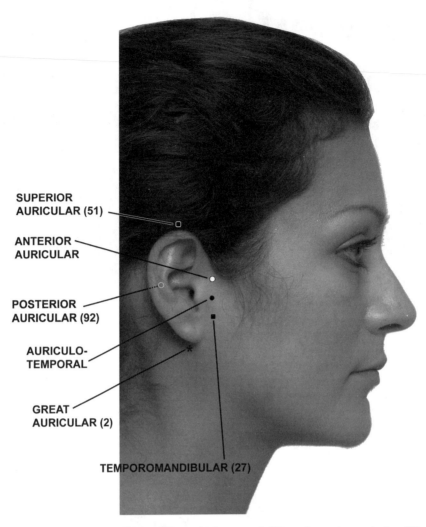

**FIGURE 11.5** The triad of the temporomandibular (27), auriculotemporal (U), and anterior auricular (U) acupoints, which are secondary, tertiary, and nonspecific, respectively. Also shown are the great auricular (2), superior auricular (51), and posterior auricular (92) points, useful for the treatment of TMJ. The posterior auricular point cannot actually be seen in this photo because it is obscured by the ear; the point is at the site where the skin of the ear meets the scalp.

includes three additional points discussed later in the context of temporomandibular joint syndrome. The Auriculotemporal and Anterior Auricular points were not included in Dung's original research establishing the sequence of the acupoints, so they are specified as unnumbered. They are nonetheless clinically quite important in treating conditions of the face and head.

It should be noted that the derivation of fibers of the Superior Auricular (51) acupoint is controversial; the point is listed here because its afferent innervation most likely comes from the mandibular division of the trigeminal (V) nerve while the efferent fibers to the superior auricular muscle come from the facial (VII) nerve. See also the discussion of this point in Chapter 5 and the introductory paragraph to the topic of acupoints of the facial nerve (VII) below.

The Mentalis (U) derives from a pair of tiny nerves that course beneath the lip. It is rarely used. The Masseter (30) acupoint overlies the masseter muscle at the mandib-

ular angle. The nerve passes over the mandibular notch to enter the inner surface of the muscle. The masseter nerve is small and deep inside the muscle and, because it is a muscular rather than a cutaneous nerve, contains afferent and efferent fibers. The Temporalis (59) acupoint is similar to the Masseter (30). The temporalis nerve is a muscular nerve branch of V3 that enters its muscle (the temporalis) deep to it. It is approximately the same size as the masseter.

### 11.3.2 ACUPOINTS OF THE SPINAL ACCESSORY NERVE (XI)

The spinal accessory nerve (XI) is located on the shoulder and is properly considered in the next chapter. However, because of some overlap between conditions of the head and face and those of the neck and shoulder (e.g., "tension" headache), points of the spinal accessory nerve are often used in treating headache and other conditions of the head and face. Please consult the next chapter for more details about this important nerve.

### 11.3.3 ACUPOINTS OF THE FACIAL NERVE (VII)

The facial nerve is a mixed nerve, having afferent fibers for the special sense of taste (which, as mentioned earlier, more distally course with V3), preganglionic parasympathetic nerves, and efferent fibers to the skeletal muscles of facial expression. Whether VII has afferent nerve fibers for general sensation is an academic uncertainty. Most anatomists agree that afferent fibers for the muscles of facial expression derive from V despite scant cadaver proof that branches of VII join branches of V and despite the presence of pain in patients suffering Bell's palsy, which is generally thought to be a disease of VII alone.

One would think that acupoints along the facial nerve would be important with respect to acupuncture because the nerve forms superficial neuromuscular attachments entering the muscles from the external surface. Nevertheless, they very seldom become detectable because of the small size of the tiny nerve branches as they divide to innervate at least 20 known muscles of facial expression. These acupoints can be designated by their associated muscles, such as Orbicularis; Depressor Labii Inferioris; Zygomaticus Major; Risorius; Levator Labii Superioris; Alaeque Nasi; Orbicularis Oculi; and Frontalis. Of these, only the Frontalis (100) is an acupoint identified in the progression of pain as described by Dung's original work. As discussed previously, the existence of afferent fibers in the facial nerve is controversial, and many authorities believe the afferent fibers from these muscles actually belong to the trigeminal nerve. Figure 11.6 shows some of these muscles and their associated acupoints, which can be useful in treating Bell's palsy.

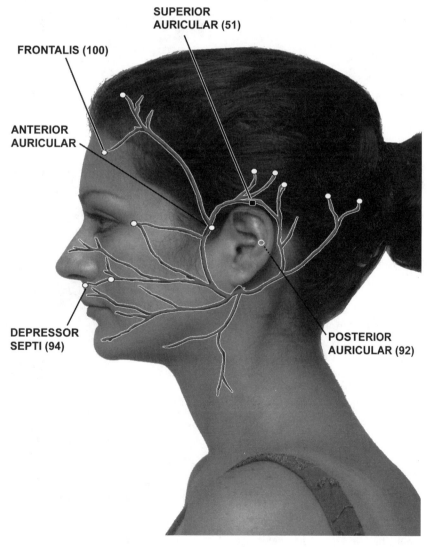

**FIGURE 11.6** Some of the branches of the facial (VII) nerve forming neuromuscular attachments with muscles of facial expression.

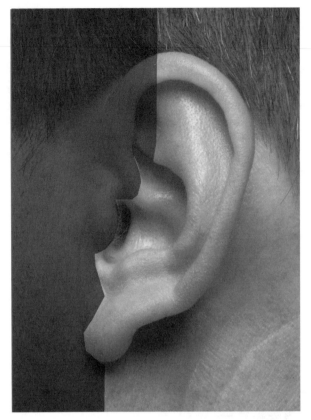

**FIGURE 11.7a** Cutaneous innervation of the ear region: distribution in and around the ear of the trigeminal nerve (shaded area).

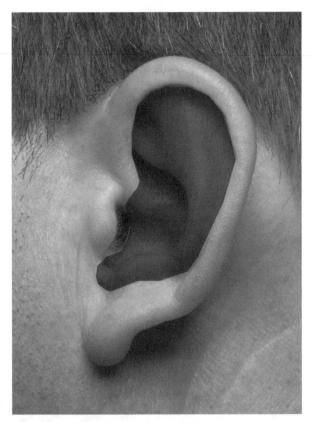

**FIGURE 11.7b** Cutaneous innervation of the ear region (continued): distribution in the ear of the facial nerve (shaded area).

### 11.3.4  ACUPOINTS OF THE GLOSSOPHARYNGEAL (IX) AND VAGUS (X) NERVES

These two cranial nerves are relevant only to *auriculopuncture*, acupuncture in the ear used primarily to treat addictions to drugs (including tobacco), obesity, and pain in other parts of the body. At first glance, a physiologic explanation for these effects may be hard to fathom. The ear is unique, however, in that it is innervated by four cranial nerves — V, VII, IX, and X — and the cervical spinal nerves (see Figure 11.7a through Figure 11.7e). This is the only structure in our body with so many different nerves congregated in so small an area. The complexity of the innervation and the small size of the region have prevented the authors from studying this area extensively and the only discussion of auriculopuncture in this text, in reference to the treatment of addictions, follows later in this chapter.

## 11.4  ACUPUNCTURE AND PAINFUL CONDITIONS OF THE FACE AND HEAD

In a patient with pain in the face and head, the practitioner should first evaluate acupoints remote from the head region to establish a systemic pain level; the acupoints in

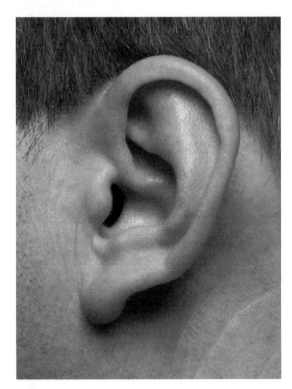

**FIGURE 11.7c** Cutaneous innervation of the ear region (continued): distribution of the glossopharyngeal nerve in the external canal in the ear (shaded area).

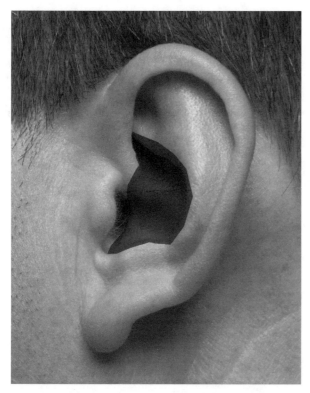

**FIGURE 11.7d** Cutaneous innervation of the ear region (continued): distribution in the ear of the vagus nerve (shaded area).

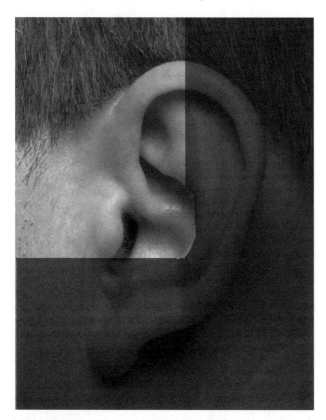

**FIGURE 11.7e** Cutaneous innervation of the ear region (continued): distribution in and around the ear of the cervical spinal nerves (shaded area).

the head will give an indication of specific conditions. The clinician should consider the overall pain level as an indication of the likelihood of success and, if that likelihood is high, should target specific passive points in the face and head and primary points throughout the body. Aside from the systemic pain quantification level, the clinician should also consider the length of time the patient has suffered from the condition because longstanding pain in the face and head is less likely to benefit from acupuncture. A corollary to this statement is that primary care physicians should consider acupuncture early in the treatment of headache patients. Application of this approach, and exceptions to it, are discussed next.

Dung's earlier studies[1] indicated that 9% of his series of acupuncture patients present with a chief complaint of pain in the head or facial area. For example, in 1995, out of 881 new patients, 74 complained of pain in the face or head, and of those 69 described their pain as "headache." Much less common presentations included neuralgia, tumor, post-herpetic pain, Bell's palsy, and facial paralysis. Whatever the description of the condition, however, all pain in this region can be categorized as trigeminal or nontrigeminal in origin. This chapter will describe trigeminal and nontrigeminal pain separately.

One kind of headache, described as occipital or back headache, arises from the cervical spinal nerves as well as the spinal accessory nerve (XI) and will be discussed in the following chapter. These headaches are also sometimes referred to as "tension" headaches, although this somewhat loose term can also be applied to trigeminal headaches.

## 11.5 TRIGEMINAL PAIN

Pain described as migraine headache, sinusitis headache, tension headache, cluster headache, trigeminal neuralgia, post-herpetic neuralgia, temporomandibular joint syndrome, and postoperative facial pain can arise from branches of the trigeminal (V) nerve. Of all these types of head pain, migraine is the most frequently seen. Migraine headache has a number of clinical presentations. It can inflict patients from 15 to 80 years old. Pain can be on one or both sides of the head. Some patients have a headache once a year; others have one daily. The severity of migraine can be from relatively mild to very extreme, including nausea, vomiting, and aura. The duration of symptoms may vary from a few months to more than 30 years. Individuals' symptoms vary so widely that one could say that no such entity as a typical migraine headache exists. Migraines vary not only from patient to patient but also, in an individual patient, from episode to episode.

Migraine sufferers typically spend years with pharmacological therapy before seeking acupuncture treatment. This is unfortunate because migraine is quite responsive to acupuncture in its early stages, but as time passes and the patient's pain level increases under the influence of continuing headaches, the headaches become less responsive to any treatment, including acupuncture. A migraine patient with a pain sensitivity of five or less can usually get at least temporary relief in three to four sessions of acupuncture. After this relief is achieved, it is necessary to repeat the treatments as often as necessary to keep the patient completely free of headaches for a month's time. This is accomplished by having three to five sessions in the first series of treatments and then waiting 4 days to have the patient come back for the next session.

If the patient has not had a headache after the 4-day lapse, needles are placed and the patient is told to come back in a week. If the patient remains headache free after that week's wait, needles are placed and the patient is told to wait 10 days to return for a final session. If at any point after the first series, the patient returns having had a new headache, the process is begun again, with three to five sessions as in the first series. If this is successfully undertaken, it is uncommon for these individuals' headaches to recur.

### 11.5.1 MIGRAINE CASE STUDIES

Marsha, a 31-year-old female, is an illustrative case. She had been suffering three headaches a week requiring emergency department injections for relief when she first presented to the acupuncture clinic. During her menstrual periods, severe dysmenorrhea would trigger her headaches; bright light and loud noises were other triggers. Her headaches usually began and always ended on the left side. She had tried chiropractic manipulation, which brought only temporary relief, and reflexology, which had no effect. Her systemic pain sensitivity was estimated to be three degrees because she had only primary points in the passive phase outside her head and neck.

The primary acupoints in the face, Infraorbital (19) and Supraorbital (23), and neck, Great Auricular (2), Spinal Accessory-I (3), and Greater Occipital (7), were very tender to palpation. The secondary acupoints, Temporomandibular (27), Cervical Plexus (28), Masseter (30), Lesser Occipital (34), Mental (50), and Superior Auricular (51), were also tender. Even a few tertiary acupoints, such as the Temporalis (59), Pterion (72), and Bregma (75) were slightly tender. The appearance of passive acupoints in the head and neck region is very typical of headache sufferers, even in the early stages of headache development.

Marsha's headaches were easily managed in 10 treatments. In the first session, she was placed in the supine position and needles were placed in each of 28 accessible primary acupoints: Supraorbital (23), Infraorbital (19), Great Auricular (2), Greater Occipital (7), Spinal Accessory-I (3), Lateral Antebrachial Cutaneous (9), Deep Radial-I (1), Superficial Radial (12), Lateral Pectoral (17), Iliotibial-I (18), Saphenous-I (4), Common Peroneal-I (24), Tibial-I (6), and Deep Peroneal (5). These points are listed in the order in which they would likely be needled.

Note that the Greater Occipital acupoint, although posterior, is accessible from the front of the body by reaching behind the neck. Also recall that short needles (0.5 in.) would be used in the face and head, long ones (1.5 to 2.0 in.) below the waist, and medium ones (1 in.) in the rest of the body, specifically, in this instance, the arms, neck, shoulders, and the Lateral Pectoral acupoint. Consistency in this regard greatly simplifies the process of removing and sorting needles for reuse.

When she returned for her second session 48 hours later, Marsha had not experienced any more headaches. She was treated in the prone position with needles placed in the primary acupoints. Although the individual sites were not recorded, a characteristic pattern would be:

- Great Auricular (2)
- Greater Occipital (7)
- Spinal Accessory-I (3)
- Dorsal Scapular (13)
- Infraspinatus (8)
- Posterior Cutaneous of T6 (21)
- Spinous Process of T7 (20)
- Lateral Antebrachial Cutaneous (9)
- Deep Radial-I (1)
- Superficial Radial (12)
- Posterior Cutaneous of L2 (15)
- Superior Cluneal (14)
- Posterior Cutaneous of L5 (22)
- Inferior Gluteal (16)
- Iliotibial-I (18)
- Saphenous-I (4)
- Lateral Popliteal (11)
- Common Peroneal-I (24)
- Tibial-I (6)
- Sural-I (10)

Two days later, as is typical of these patients on their third visit, she was placed in the sitting position and all the tender points in her face and head area — primary, secondary, or tertiary — were needled. Practitioners should exercise caution when needling sitting patients because syncope is a frequent complication of acupuncture in this position. (Chapter 8 includes a discussion of avoiding this complication and Chapter 9, a discussion of managing it if it should occur.)

Marsha had a total of 10 treatments with two additional headaches occurring during the course of treatment, but eventually the headaches completely disappeared. The subsequent treatments after the first three were essentially repeating cycles of the treatment series described previously, with periodic breaks to see if the headaches would reemerge. (Note that she was treated with a different protocol from that described earlier for keeping a patient headache free for a month's time.)

This course of therapy is typical for patients with conditions in the face and head. Bill, a 36-year-old auto dealer estimated to have four degrees of systemic sensitivity, was relieved of his migraine headaches after only five treatments that varied little from those administered to Marsha. He had undergone a complete work-up of his headaches and been given medications to abort them, but his headaches typically came on during sleep, awakening him too late in their development for the medications to be effective. Males respond to acupuncture treatments for migraine better than females. Most migraines are reported by females; less than 30% of migraine sufferers seen in the clinic have been males.

Sharon, a 50-year-old female, was a solid four degrees systemically when she was first seen in the clinic. Because she had a higher sensitivity than Marsha's, a number of secondary acupoints were added during treatment to the primary ones throughout the body. Because she had more tender points in the face and head, more points were needled there as well. In her face and head, five secondary points (Temporomandibular, Cervical Plexus, Masseter, Lesser Occipital, and Mental), three tertiary (Temporalis, Pterion, and Zygomaticofacial), and two nonspecific points (Nasion and Lacrimal) were included in the treatments. Many points were needled because Sharon perceived slight sensation, although not enough to be described as tenderness, when these more minor points were palpated gently. After the fourth treatment, the headaches disappeared completely; five more treatments were then done to keep the headaches at bay for the requisite 30 days.

The patients reviewed represent success stories because of their low pain sensitivities. More often, headache sufferers present with higher pain sensitivities, often in the seven to nine degree range. Lois, a 26-year-old female with a pain sensitivity of six, is an example of a treatment failure. She had a total of 57 acupuncture treatments and during those treatments had one 4-month, headache-free period, but ultimately stopped coming for treatment. She had suffered migraines since the age of 9 or 10, illustrating another point about headaches: those that are long-standing are more intractable to treatment regardless of pain sensitivity.

Bill, a 75-year-old retired rancher, illustrates another point. Acupuncture affected his headaches somewhat, but failed to resolve them completely, despite the fact that Bill had a pain sensitivity of only four degrees. His case is typical in that older persons are more difficult to treat for headaches, regardless of pain sensitivity.

The authors have anecdotally noticed an association among migraine headache, low diastolic blood pressure, and dysmenorrhea, suggesting that hormonal influences may play a role in the causation of migraine and its response to acupuncture. The association seems strong enough to warrant further academic study.

The authors are convinced that migraine can be managed easily and effectively if its duration is less than a year in a patient with a pain level of four degrees or less. Headaches with duration of 1 or 2 years in a patient with a pain level between five and seven degrees still can be managed to a limited extent, but with a strong possibility that relapses will eventually occur. At the extreme, patients with pain levels greater than seven degrees who have suffered headaches longer than 4 years cannot be effectively managed. Unfortunately, because headache sufferers often consider acupuncture as a last resort, they present at the clinic late in the course of their disease — too late for acupuncture to be of much benefit. This fact highlights the importance of primary care physicians' use of acupuncture; they are the practitioners most likely to see patients early in the course of their illnesses and thus have the greatest opportunity to intervene successfully.

### 11.5.2 SINUS HEADACHES

Next to migraine, headache associated with sinusitis is the second most common type of pain in the head region, although far fewer cases of sinus headache than of migraine present to the acupuncture clinic. These headaches are caused by sinus infection or inflammation in the frontal regions of the skull innervated by the trigeminal distribution, in reaction to environmental allergens. Not everyone with sinus allergies will develop headaches. This is an unusual application in that acupuncture seems to alleviate the underlying condition rather than simply the painful manifestation of the condition. For this reason, the treatment of sinus allergy is treated separately later in this chapter, outside the context of painful conditions.

However, it is relevant to point out that the treatment of sinus headache is fairly similar to treatment of other headaches, such as migraine, with the addition of a few additional acupoints to the migraine treatment regimen. Pain sensitivity in patients with sinus headache is found to be relatively low, usually less than six degrees and often in the three-degree range. However, the response to treatment seems independent of this sensitivity, almost certainly because treatment of the underlying sinus condition is mediated through the parasympathetic nervous system, which is independent of nociception. Sinus headaches, like other allergy manifestations in the face and head, are usually very easy to manage and eliminate.

### 11.5.3 TENSION AND CLUSTER HEADACHES

Tension and cluster headaches are placed together for discussion for three reasons: (1) they are not commonly seen; (2) both types of headache appear to affect males more than females; and (3) these patients generally have low pain levels and their headaches are usually easy to manage. Once managed, these headaches rarely, if ever,

**TABLE 11.1**
**Biostatistical Profile of Patients with Trigeminal Neuralgia**

| Year | Case # | Age | Sex | Etiology | Side | Division | Duration | Degree | Sessions | Results |
|------|--------|-----|-----|----------|------|----------|----------|--------|----------|---------|
| 1990 | 1 | 12 | Female | Unknown | Right | Maxillary | 2 months | 7 | 7 | Good |
| 1990 | 2 | 63 | Male | Postherpetic neuralgia[a] | Right | Maxillary | 10 years | 5 | 9 | Pain reduced |
| 1992 | 1 | 44 | Female | Dental work | Left | Maxillary | 5 years | 9 | 2 | Quit; needles painful |
| 1992 | 2 | 71 | Female | Unknown | Right | Maxillary | 5 years | 8 | 7 | Quit |
| 1993 | 1 | 73 | Female | Unknown | Left | Maxillary | 10 years | 10 | 12 | Improved |
| 1993 | 2 | 84 | Female | Dental work | Right | Maxillary | 6 months | 8 | 7 | Improved |
| 1993 | 3 | 53 | Male | Dental work | Right | Maxillary | 2 years | 3 | 3 | Good |
| 1994 | 1 | 55 | Female | Unknown | Left | Maxillary | 2 years | 5 | 5 | No change |
| 1994 | 2 | 73 | Female | Unknown | Left | Maxillary | Unknown | 12 | 4 | No change |
| 1994 | 3 | 63 | Female | Dental work | Right | Mandibular | 6 months | 8 | 4 | Improved |
| 1994 | 4 | 80 | Female | Dental work | Right | Maxillary | 20 years | 9 | 28 | Modest improvement |
| 1995 | 1 | 46 | Female | Car crash | Right | Mandibular | 11 years | 4 | 3 | No change |
| 1995 | 2 | 74 | Female | Unknown | Left | Mandibular | 5 years | 7 | 17 | Possibly improved |
| 1995 | 3 | 51 | Female | Dental work | Right | Maxillary | 7 years | 5 | 26 | Improved |
| 1996 | 1 | 75 | Female | Dental work | Left | Mandibular | 3 months | 5 | 3 | Excellent |
| 1996 | 2 | 64 | Female | Unknown | Left | Maxillary | 3 years | 8 | 10 | No change |

[a] Case #2 in 1990 was diagnosed by the first treating physician as having trigeminal neuralgia, but he later recalled at the acupuncture clinic that he had suffered an episode of herpes zoster 10 years earlier, shortly before his headaches started.

recur. The anecdotal associations with tension headaches include prior neck injury (cervical strain or sprain); relatively low blood pressure; dysmenorrhea; sleep disorders; and, of course, psychologically stressful situations such as abuse. These conditions are also associated with pain in the neck and shoulders (described in the next chapter). Cluster headaches are rarely seen and then almost always in males; their response depends on pain sensitivity. Treatment for cluster and tension headaches is essentially the same as for migraines, with the addition of points in the neck and shoulders as indicated for pain in that anatomical region (described in the next chapter).

### 11.5.4 NEURALGIC PAIN

Neuralgic pain affecting the trigeminal nerve can affect the face and head. Two neuralgias occur in the head and face: trigeminal neuralgia (tic douloureux) and post-herpetic neuralgia. Both occur along divisions of the trigeminal nerve. Trigeminal neuralgia is perceived along areas innervated by branches of the maxillary and mandibular divisions, which innervate the areas most affected by dental work. Dental drillings have great potential to trigger the occurrence of trigeminal neuralgia in individuals with a high degree of pain sensitivity, as seen in Table 11.1, which describes 16 patients thought to have trigeminal neuralgia in author Dung's practice over a 7-year period.

On the other hand, pain produced by post-herpetic neuralgia is almost always located along the courses of the ophthalmic and maxillary divisions but not the mandibular division (an exceptional case is discussed later).

The two neuralgias have several similarities. Both tend to occur in an older population. Most sufferers have pain sensitivities between seven and ten degrees; those with four or less are unusual. Predictably, this pain is not easy to manage, with the exception of patients with a relatively short duration of suffering (less than 3 months). Once the pain has persisted for a year or more, both neuralgias are virtually impossible to manage.

### 11.5.5 TRIGEMINAL NEURALGIA (TIC DOULOUREUX)

Fortunately, tic douloureux is not often seen. As can be seen from Table 11.1, in the period of 7 years from 1990 to 1996, only a total of 16 patients with tic were treated. The authors note that in those 7 years, 87% of tic patients were females, compared to 13% males. The table illustrates that these patients are difficult to manage because they typically come for acupuncture late in the course of their disease when their pain sensitivities are high. The treatment protocol is essentially the same as for headaches, with special attention paid to the area where pain is perceived.

One example of a patient experiencing good results from acupuncture was Linda, depicted on the first line of Table 11.1. Linda's example shows that acupuncture can be beneficial to treat trigeminal neuralgia in selected cases. Because she was 12 years old, she was among the youngest patients ever seen in the clinic (children are understandably reluctant to experience needling) and her youth probably contributed to her good result. Trigeminal neuralgia is typically a disease of the elderly; for a young person to have this problem is very uncommon. Linda's pain sensitivity of seven degrees at such a young age was another surprise. She had been to several dentists and a pediatric neurologist before coming for acupuncture; she was referred by her neurologist. Her youth and short duration of symptoms (2 months) were apparently more significant for her good result than her relatively high pain sensitivity. It is unfortunate that her pain sensitivity and menstrual and pain history were not followed through subsequent years.

Ruby, a 51-year-old female depicted in the table as the third patient seen in 1995, is an example of a patient who was more difficult to manage, but who still found eventual relief with acupuncture. Between her first dental drilling at age 19 and the beginning of her neuralgia at age 44 was a long interval. She believed that her dental problem was the source of her pain because the pain was always perceived in the right upper lip over her canine tooth in the maxillary bone, a tooth that had caused her many problems and undergone several dental procedures over the years. Still, the connection was not clear because her last dental care was 7 years prior to her trying acupuncture. Because she had a pain sensitivity of only five degrees, one would think the tic would be easy to manage, but it was in fact difficult.

The tic on the right side of Ruby's face was limited to the area around the infraorbital foramen extending inferiorly to the upper lip. The pain could be triggered by mastication and conversation and episodes were intermittent and random. The pain would sometimes be mitigated without any intervention yet could just as easily be unrelenting. Ruby was anxious to try any available therapy and had already tried microvascular decompression, a technique aimed at relieving the pressure against the nerve by an adjacent blood vessel, and percutaneous injections, which can cause numbness in the nerve's distribution — both to no avail. The failure of these treatments reduced the authors' confidence in using acupuncture for her tic. Nevertheless, Ruby was resolved to try. After a total of 15 treatments between November 13 and December 27, 1995, her tic appeared to show some alleviation. The frequency of attacks and the intensity of pain lessened.

The protocol for Ruby's tic should be familiar to the reader at this point: the supine, prone, and sitting positions were used in rotation. The total number of needles given in each session incrementally increased from 30 in each of the first three treatments to 55 in each of the last three. Only primary acupoints were used outside the head and neck regions. Every passive acupoint available on the face and over the entire skull was needled at least one time during the 15 treatments. Twice, four needles were placed through the mucous membrane covering the right maxillary canine tooth on the vestibular side of the oral cavity.

Acupuncture attempts began to bear some results. By January 6, 1996, when Ruby came for her 16th treatment,

she claimed that she was 75% improved. The pain was concentrated over the canine tooth. Four days later, she came for the 17th time and said that there was no more pain with chewing and talking. She was advised to wait and see and return to the clinic whenever the tic recurred. She returned 70 days later because the tic was back. She was given six more treatments concluding April 19, 1996. After that, the tic stayed dormant longer, until January 23, 1997. This time Ruby's tic was stopped after only one treatment, but she came for two more sessions and, by January 28, 1997, she had received 26 treatments. This appears to have resolved her tic permanently because she has not returned for more treatment since that time.

As can be seen from the table, because many patients who are elderly and have high degrees of sensitivity do not receive total relief from acupuncture. Many, however, are helped.

### 11.5.6 Post-Herpetic Neuralgia

Post-herpetic neuralgia is far more common than trigeminal neuralgia and can occur practically anywhere in the body. Cases that occur outside the head region will be discussed in other chapters; attention here will be focused on post-herpetic neuralgia in the head. Like tic, post-herpetic pain is not an easy condition to manage. The manageability depends on two factors: duration of the condition and the patient's pain sensitivity. A number of patients with post-herpetic pain who have a pain sensitivity of five degrees or lower have been seen in the clinic shortly after activation of the virus; these patients have good results from acupuncture.

John, a 77-year-old Air Force retiree, is an example of an acupuncture patient obtaining good results for this condition. John came to the clinic because of pain in the left side of his forehead extending to the temporal and parietal regions. The pain was caused by a herpes infection of the ophthalmic division of his trigeminal nerve that occurred in October 1995. Physicians at an Air Force hospital had treated him for the skin (mostly scalp) lesions, which healed rather quickly in a couple of weeks. The pain lingered after the lesions resolved, and his doctors told him that it might take months for the pain to subside. He waited for almost 5 months and the pain persisted. His doctors again told him that nothing more could be done for the pain; they did not prescribe any pain medication. He was told to be patient and that the pain would subside on its own. When he first presented at the clinic for acupuncture treatments, his pain sensitivity was assessed at six degrees.

John was first treated in a supine position, with needles placed in primary acupoints throughout the entire body and about 25 more needles placed over the scalp where he perceived the pain. These needles are typically placed at the periphery of any visible lesion, generally encircling it, rather than directly into it. The second treatment was given after placing him in the prone position. Again, needles were placed in each of the accessible primary points and some 25 more were placed in nonspecific points in the scalp area. The third treatment was administered with John in a sitting position; primary, secondary, tertiary, and nonspecific points on the face, scalp, neck, and upper limbs were needled. The fourth treatment was given with him lying on his right side, and the fifth was the same as the second, with John in the prone position.

A total of five treatments was provided as a series within 10 days. Then a 1-week waiting period was set, after which the patient returned for another series of three more treatments duplicating the first three of the first series. The pain began to show signs of diminishing as the frequency and severity of attacks were decreasing. The third and last series of three treatments was administered after another 1-week waiting period. The last and 11th treatment was given on April 25, 1996. By then the patient stated that he had been free of pain for almost a week.

Richard, the 63-year-old father of the physician who referred him for acupuncture only 6 weeks after an active herpes activation, also benefited from acupuncture for his subsequent neuralgia. This case is highly unusual in that it is the only case ever seen by the authors in which the herpes infection involved all three divisions of the trigeminal nerve. Richard experienced pain over the entire side of his scalp and face, even inside his cheek. The pain interfered with his sleep.

Richard was found to have a pain sensitivity of five degrees. The treating acupuncturist was optimistic and predicted that his pain could be stopped in six to eight treatments. The first treatment was administered while he was in the supine position using the primary acupoints, including those in the face. Because he had a long distance to travel to the clinic, Richard stayed overnight and returned the next day for his second treatment. He was very happy because he had enjoyed the best night's sleep in more than a month. The second treatment was done when he was in the prone position with only primary acupoints needled. One day later, he came for the third session. He said that the pain flared up somewhat after the second treatment; this illustrates the point that too intensive treatments in too short a period of time can flare the sensation of pain. Thus, he was advised to return home and wait for 3 days before trying any more acupuncture. The third treatment included needles on the mental and masseter points bilaterally. Many nonspecific points on the face and scalp were used because these points were passive.

Richard returned to receive his fourth treatment, similar to the first but with extra needles placed in a number of nonspecific points. At his fifth visit 4 days later, his post-herpetic pain was still present with slightly less intensity. The supine position was used again for the fifth ses-

sion to repeat the protocol for the fourth. When Richard returned 3 days later, the pain was substantially diminished. On his last visit a few days later, he said that he was practically free of pain and sleeping well. He was placed in the supine position to take care of acupoints on the face and the ventral side of the body. He was advised to return in a week if he still had pain but did not return for further treatment.

John and Richard were unusual cases in that their pain was completely relieved with acupuncture. Other patients with advanced age, high pain sensitivities, and long-standing duration of disease should be informed about their poor likelihood of complete success with acupuncture prior to beginning treatments. Many of these patients will have some degree of relief but only a minority will have total success.

### 11.5.7 TEMPOROMANDIBULAR JOINT SYNDROME

The temporomandibular joint is innervated by the trigeminal nerve, as are the muscles of mastication (by V3, the mandibular division of the nerve). The pathophysiology of the painful disorder referred to as "temporomandibular joint syndrome," or "TMJ," is not very well understood and even the existence of the syndrome is controversial. TMJ patients seen in the clinic are six times more likely to be female and most are between the ages of 35 and 55.

Six acupoints are located around the ear, as shown in Figure 11.5:

1. Great Auricular (2), a primary acupoint
2. Temporomandibular (27), secondary
3. Auriculotemporal (U), tertiary
4. Anterior Auricular (U), nonspecific
5. Superior Auricular (51), secondary
6. Posterior Auricular (92), nonspecific

If the examiner finds, in assessing sensitivity, that the Great Auricular and Temporomandibular points are passive but the other four are not, then it is likely that the patient will not manifest symptoms of TMJ. However, if only one more of the other four points is passive, the patient will most likely exhibit symptoms. Many TMJ patients will have tenderness in all six of these points. It follows from this discussion that virtually all TMJ patients will have a pain sensitivity of four degrees or higher, and in fact no TMJ patient has been seen in our clinic with a pain sensitivity less than four. Therefore, TMJ in general is not an easy problem to manage, and sufferers will most likely have incomplete or temporary relief at best, while a minority, especially those who present soon after the onset of symptoms, will have complete relief. Steffany T. is one example of the latter.

Steffany, a 17-year-old high school student, wrote out her complete medical history before coming to the clinic. She stated:

> My neck, shoulders, and throat are always tight. My throat gets real tight when I sing, talk, or chew. My ears ache as if I have "swimmer's ear." I always have a headache at the temples and in between my eyes. My temples and the upper right side of my jaw are tender to the touch. My left side pops at the joint, but it doesn't bother me as much as the right side does. My bottom teeth feel like they are going to fall out! When I eat soft food, talk very little, and don't sing, it helps! I constantly take Ibuprofen, Tylenol, and Excedrin to relieve the pain. Ice packs and Mineral Ice are great to use while the pain killers are kicking in. Hurts when I whistle and for some unknown reason I am always crying. These symptoms have been going on for about 3 years. I have been to see:
>
> (1) Oral dental surgeon — took out my wisdom teeth, thinking they were pressing on a nerve
>
> (2) Two chiropractors — couldn't find anything wrong
>
> (3) Orthodontist — prescribed mouthpiece
>
> (4) Regular dentist — nothing, possibly tension

The youngest patient with TMJ ever seen in the clinic, Steffany was assessed to have a pain sensitivity of six degrees. Acupuncture treatments for her turned out to have an excellent result, most likely because of her young age. The first treatment was administered with the patient in the supine position using 24 primary points, plus two needles in the Temporomandibular and Auriculotemporal acupoints around each ear. Two days later, she came for the second treatment and indicated that her symptoms were somewhat reduced. She was asked if she knew her blood pressure and she stated explicitly that it was 93/70. She also affirmed that she suffered from menstrual cramping. The authors suspect that these two factors — relatively low blood pressure and dysmenorrhea — are associated with high pain sensitivity levels and especially a tendency to pain in the upper portion of the body.

For the second treatment, Steffany was placed in the prone position for needling in the primary points on the dorsal surface of the body, along with the same two points in front of each ear as in the first treatment. She came for the third visit 2 days later and was then treated while she was in the sitting position with needles placed in the primary and secondary acupoints on the head, neck, shoulders, and other parts of the upper extremities, along with the same two points in front of each ear. She was told to wait for 1 week and then return for one or two more sessions if she was still experiencing symptoms.

She came for a fourth visit a week later; at that time she complained only of slight discomfort around the left ear. She was then treated lying on her right side so that the left ear would be easily accessible. Accessible primary points were needled along with four points around the left ear: Auriculotemporal (U); Temporomandibular (27); Superior Auricular (51); and Posterior Auricular (92). She was told to return if the pain relapsed, and she did 4 months later. At that fifth visit, she associated the relapse of her TMJ problem with chewing and some jumping exercises. She also said that sweating seemed to ease the pain momentarily. Over the next 5 days, three more treatments were given with the same protocol described for the first three visits. She had complete relief after a total of seven treatments. It is possible that she might have needed only four visits or less if her pain sensitivity had been five degrees or less. Incidentally, Steffany related that she cried less after the acupuncture treatments.

TMJ does not seem to be a consequence of systemic disease but rather is local in nature; thus, it often appears unilaterally in the beginning. In patients with only unilateral pain, treatment is more likely to be successful; those with bilateral pain have more established disease and thus are harder to treat. Most TMJ cases have mixed results. TMJ is easier to manage than migraine, tic douloureux, and post-herpetic neuralgia, using the six points around the ear as described above.

### 11.5.8 POSTOPERATIVE FACIAL PAIN

Surgery such as that to remove neoplasms or plastic surgery can result in pain in the face for some patients. It is not uncommon for plastic surgery to produce pain. A few cases seen in the clinic had pain behind the ears and extending to the neck. Some of these patients did not even recognize the pain as a consequence of the surgery. Facial pain after plastic surgery, in general, is not difficult to stop because most patients come to be seen soon after the surgery. It is a pain of an acute nature and is therefore relatively easy to manage. Patients who develop facial pain after plastic surgery often have pain levels of four degrees or higher, suggesting that postoperative pain after these procedures does not occur in lower degree patients. Treatment of this pain is identical to that for headache with an emphasis in using acupoints around the ears and other locations on the face where the pain is perceived.

### 11.6 BELL'S PALSY

Bell's palsy, also known as facial paralysis, is a disease of the facial (VII) cranial nerve. It was first reported by Dr. Charles Bell, a British neurologist, more than 150 years ago.[2] Extensive writings about the disease can be found in the medical literature.[3,4] Much is known about the disease but not much is available to treat it. For this reason, it is not uncommon for patients with facial paralysis to seek acupuncture treatment. Sometimes, a patient will complain of pain occurring in the paralyzed area, generally some time after the face became paralyzed. The disease is self-limited, meaning that it will eventually resolve on its own without medical treatment.

The facial nerve contains efferent (motor) and afferent (sensory) fibers. There are two types of efferent fibers in the facial nerve: one controls the muscles of facial expression and the other is the collection of autonomic nerves that control secretion of tears and saliva. The afferent fibers are the nerves for special senses that innervate the taste buds on the tongue. Anatomically, the facial nerve is not known to contain afferent fibers for the general sensation of pain. Thus, it is a puzzle why some patients with Bell's palsy should have facial pain. One plausible explanation is that trigeminal nerve may be involved, but the nature of such a potential involvement is not known.

Epidemiologically, Bell's palsy occurs in 22.8 persons out of a population of 100,000 annually, or 228 per million.[5] In a 15-year period in our clinic serving a city of 1 million, only 26 Bell's palsy patients were seen. Because paralysis is efferent in nature, acupuncture would be expected to be of little value, and then primarily for the occasional accompanying pain. These cases have tended to be difficult and to have mixed results. The result does not appear to be correlated with the pain sensitivity level, but may be more a matter of the degree of damage to the facial nerve. Several examples are given to illustrate this puzzling disorder.

One is Wendy, a 65-year-old housewife. Wendy came for the first time after experiencing Bell's palsy for 7 years. The condition was painless but the paralysis seemed to be progressing. Her main complaint was that liquids would drool out of the right corner of her mouth as she drank, and she would experience numbness in that area as well. Through careful observation of her face when she smiled, an observer could see an asymmetrical contortion, in that the right labial commissure was lower than the left. She was the first case of Bell's palsy seen in the clinic and there was little confidence that she could be helped with acupuncture. She was treated 11 times during the first month of treatment and then asked to wait for 2 weeks.

When she returned, she reported improved sleep and the numbness at the right corner of her mouth had disappeared. Six weeks later, she came back because she felt that the palsy was relapsing. Five more treatments were provided. Her symptoms subsided for another 6 months, but then she came for an 18th treatment to reduce symptoms of drooling and numbness. Another three treatments were given before her symptoms cleared. At the same time, she complained of pain in the left lower back. The low back pain was taken care of in a few treatments. Thereafter, she kept returning for the same low back pain

and pain in other locations, but never complained of the Bell's palsy again.

Helen, a 66-year-old female, is Wendy's sister-in-law. When she developed Bell's palsy, she sought acupuncture immediately because of her familiarity with Wendy's experience. (Given the low incidence of the condition and the lack of a blood relationship between Helen and Wendy, the likelihood of this happening to two similarly associated individuals should be exceedingly low; this suggests that the condition may have an infectious or environmental cause.) Helen first came to the clinic 2 days after being diagnosed with the illness. At the time of her arrival, she was taking antiinflammatory drugs. The entire left side of her face was paralyzed and she experienced severe accompanying pain, particularly along the left nasolabial groove.

With the experience gained from treating Wendy, the authors concluded that at least 20 acupoints in the face could be used to treat Helen's Bell's palsy. This number was derived from the fact that about 20 muscles in the face are innervated by branches of the facial nerve, as shown in Figure 11.6. Each of the muscles should have an acupoint formed by the neuromuscular attachment of the nerve branches. Locating these acupoints precisely is difficult or impossible: each facial nerve has five major branches and each of these divides into a number of smaller nerve twigs to enter the muscles; each twig is too small to be dissected with an unaided eye.

Because the acupoints cannot be located precisely, needles were inserted in a nonspecific manner. Each treatment consisted of needling primary acupoints along with 10 additional secondary, tertiary, and nonspecific points on each side of the face. For instance, four needles were placed along the nasolabial groove because of perceived pain in that area. Four needles were also placed around the orbital rim of left eye because the patient could not move that eye. The supine, prone, and sitting positions were used in rotation.

By the time Helen came for the sixth treatment, the symptoms of the palsy had almost completely subsided. She was then treated for other problems: knee pain and bilateral carpal tunnel syndrome. She continued to be treated for these conditions for a total of 25 visits; until that time her palsy had not relapsed and she was free of any Bell's palsy symptoms, such as numbness, drooling, tearing, and facial asymmetry. Her case indicates that treating Bell's palsy with acupuncture immediately after symptoms appear stands a good chance of success. Even though most cases are self-limited, most cases in the clinic have been difficult to treat because the patients came months or years after symptoms developed. Compliance has been an important issue with these patients because the disfigurement and functional impairment of facial paralysis make patients impatient to achieve quick results. Most likely, because the palsy results from nerve destruction, acupuncture stimulates regeneration of the nerve, a slow process as the axon regrows through its myelin sheath from the proximal uninjured portion of the nerve. These patients require a number of acupuncture treatments to achieve relief.

An alternative hypothesis for the paralysis associated with Bell's palsy is that the efferent nerves are not injured at all; rather, the afferent nerves carrying proprioceptive signals are involved. This would explain the efficacy of acupuncture in the treatment of paralysis because, theoretically, the needles could be stimulating the proprioceptive afferent fibers. As we have said, we do not believe that acupuncture can affect efferent fibers.

Earl, a 64-year-old real estate broker, is the only patient seen at the authors' clinic with Bell's palsy on both sides of the face (not simultaneously). He came for the first time about 3 months after the onset of symptoms. The paralysis occurred in the left side of the face first. After 12 treatments in 6 weeks that used the same protocol as that for Helen, he was completely free of symptoms. Two years later, he returned with Bell's palsy on the right side of his face; he could not close his right eye completely. The duration of paralysis on the right had been 6 weeks before he decided to come for acupuncture. The right side was more difficult to treat than the left. By the 25th treatment, he was able to close his eye tighter. Thereafter, he came once every 4 to 6 days because he still had some numbness in the right corner of his mouth. Numbness is always the last sensation to resolve and harder to manage than pain itself; this may be related to the fact that fibers carrying the sensation of numbness are larger than those for pain. For Earl, the numbness took another 2 months to subside. He had a total of 38 treatments.

## 11.7 SINUS ALLERGY

As previously stated, the mechanism by which acupuncture affects sinus secretions seems to be related to interconnections between the fibers of V2 and the parasympathetic fibers originating from the superior salivatory nucleus within the brain. These parasympathetic fibers are thought to regulate the secretions of the sinus cavity. Probably as a result of this mechanism of action, the response of sinus patients to acupuncture is independent of the pain sensitivity level.

Most sinusitis patients can be successfully treated in three to six sessions. The relief is not permanent, but usually lasts through the current allergy season and sometimes for years. Patients sensitive to multiple allergens may need to be treated several times throughout the year. Of course, the treating physician should investigate avoidable sources of allergens such as household pets and the use of wood heating. Additionally, the physician should keep in mind that just as different individuals respond differently to various antiallergy medications, so do they

respond differently to different combinations of medications and acupuncture. For some, acupuncture alone may make them more comfortable; for others, medications alone may be a better solution and, for still others, some combination of the two is the best choice. Acupuncture in this setting should be considered one tool among several.

A closely related issue is that of asthma, a subject covered in Chapter 13. The conditions of sinus allergy and asthma are so similar that the acupuncture treatment for one often results in resolution of the other. The treatment for asthma can be considered an extension of the treatment for sinus allergy in that it involves the same points used in treating sinusitis with the addition of more points in the thorax. Acupuncture treatment for asthma can result in extremely gratifying improvement for a patient who has been refractory to various antiallergy regimens and frequently winds up in the hospital emergency department. The results can be so remarkable that it seems unfortunate that so many are deprived of the opportunity of this simple intervention.

The treatment of sinusitis is almost identical to the treatment of migraine. Positions are varied from supine to prone to sitting, with accessible primary points needled along with additional points in the face and head that are passive (tender). Whenever the patient's position is supine or sitting, the Supraorbital (23), Infraorbital (19), and Mental (50) points are needled, as are the Paranasal (U) ones.

The Paranasal points were discussed earlier in the chapter and depicted in Figure 11.3; their effect is suspected to be in the stimulation of postganglionic parasympathetic fibers rich in this area of the nose. The Paranasal points are the most important in this intervention. These points are quite tender to needles, so it may be advisable to needle all other points first, saving the Paranasals for last. (Generally, the face, hands, and feet are the most sensitive areas of the body and should be needled last.) When the patient is prone, the accessible primary points are needled and the Paravertebral points are added as well. These points were discussed in Chapter 8 and depicted in Figure 8.5; needles in this area are thought to cause sympathetic stimulation followed by sympathetic neurotransmitter exhaustion. (Readers may recognize the consistency of this model, in that needling the Paravertebral points is thought to reduce stress, and asthma is often clinically associated with stress.)

In the third treatment session, the patient is placed in the sitting position and needles are placed in the accessible primary and secondary points, plus the Bregma (75) and Pterion (72) points. If the patient fails to respond after the first three sessions, they are repeated with the addition of the anterior cutaneous nerves in the first two thoracic interspaces at the lateral sternal borders. If a third series is needed, the anterior cutaneous nerves in the third interspace, the Intercostobrachial (58), and the nonspecific point at the costal arch area just lateral to the xiphoid process of the sternum are also needled. Many allergy patients will have these points in the passive phase, making them easy to detect. Patients with nasal allergy problems persisting after 9 to 12 treatment sessions are unlikely to respond.

One case is illustrative: that of Shawn, a 28-year-old female secretary and bookkeeper, who described her headaches as related to her sinus allergies. She began to have sinus problems when she was in her early twenties and they continued more or less constantly, being worse in the mornings, from that time on. Her symptoms included headaches perceived in the nasion and occiput and also sore throat and coughing. She had consulted an otolaryngologist and was given nasal sprays to use; these gave only short-term relief at first, then no relief at all. On examination, only a few of Shawn's acupoints were in the passive phase, and most of those were in the head and neck. She was assessed to have a pain level of three and told it would take three sessions to relieve her headaches. She was skeptical that she would get relief so quickly after so many years of suffering.

On her first treatment, she received needles in the primary points while in the supine position. On her second visit 2 days later, she said that her frontal headache had not bothered her for about 24 hours and that her sinusitis symptoms had lessened, but that the achy feeling on the occipital protuberance was still rather outstanding. On that second visit she was placed in the prone position and needles were placed in the primary and Paravertebral points. Six extra needles were added to nonspecific points around the occipital protuberance to reduce the occipital headache. Shawn was scheduled for a third appointment 3 days later, but was not seen until more than 3 years later, when she related that her sinusitis had not bothered her since her earlier treatments. She then had two more treatments similar to the first two (sparing the occipital protuberance). She was again lost to follow-up for 5 years, when she returned to bring a friend suffering from the same condition. Gratifying cases such as Shawn's are the rule rather than the exception when treating sinus allergy. Again, this application of acupuncture suggests that primary care physicians should be able to perform these simple interventions for their patients; the risk is low and the rewards are high.

## 11.8 TINNITUS AND VERTIGO

Tinnitus and vertigo are occasionally improved with acupuncture. The physiological explanation for this improvement is not readily apparent. Sometimes even hearing loss is subjectively improved. It may be that the mechanism of action is to diminish sinus allergy symptoms. Even patients with hearing loss resulting from ototoxic drugs seem to have some improvement, but rarely is it dramatic.

When patients request acupuncture for these conditions, we are not overly optimistic about the results, but we have had enough gratifying experiences to encourage us to give every case the benefit of the doubt. We generally follow the protocol described earlier for headaches, paying special attention to the points around the ears; this is described more fully in Section 11.10 below. If no improvement is apparent after three to six treatments, acupuncture is abandoned; on the other hand, even modest improvement may be very important to some patients and their right to make their own informed decision is paramount.

## 11.9 SMOKING CESSATION, WEIGHT LOSS, AND OTHER ADDICTIONS

Addictions are included in this chapter because their therapy focuses on the ear. It would be wonderful to report that acupuncture offers promise in breaking cycles of addiction such as those associated with smoking and overeating. Unfortunately, the results are discouraging, although the few positive examples warrant continued efforts in this area. Addictions result from a complex interaction of social, psychological, and physiological factors; successful treatment requires addressing each of these factors. The authors feel that acupuncture affects the physiological addiction and, with a little creativity, can be expanded to include psychological suggestion. After all, for a person to request needle insertion to cure an addiction shows a fairly strong commitment to quitting smoking (or using smokeless tobacco, or overeating — the same discussion could apply to any addiction).

To say that acupuncture has a physiological effect is not to say that it does not have a placebo effect as well. In this setting, the placebo effect should be exploited to encourage the patient that he will be able to quit smoking as a result of the needles. Two ear staples (four for weight reduction) are left in place for 2 weeks after the acupuncture session, as will be described next; their presence is a constant reminder to the patient of his commitment to quit. To address the social aspect, the patient should be urged to keep away from places in which people smoke (e.g., nightclubs) and possibly encouraged that this might be a good time to start an exercise program (to provide an alternative activity and obtain other health benefits). It can be very difficult for a patient if another member of the household also smokes; possibly the other family member can be convinced to go outdoors to smoke. The problem lies in the relatively short treatment interval: the patient is at risk for resuming bad habits for much longer than the 2 weeks that ear staples are in place. To make the most of these 2 weeks, daily counseling and encouragement is the optimal approach. To be most effective, these acupuncture treatments should be accompanied by counseling, support groups, 12-step programs, and, possibly, medication.

When the problem is overeating, additional education should be directed to nutrition, beginning with learning to read nutrition information on food products. Weight loss begins at the grocery store. An optimal program includes daily diet recall and counseling, along with graphing daily weights. A realistic goal of 1 to 2 lb a week of weight loss should be counseled. Strict, extreme diets should be avoided in favor of incremental improvements in diet that can be sustained for life. Again, as in reducing other addictions, exercise is an important adjunct to a weight reduction program; 1 hour a day for 5 days a week of brisk walking is probably sufficient to reduce weight.

In any program to make these kinds of profound life changes, addressing the psychological component may be critical. A team psychologist can help staff and patient understand the underlying motives for addictive behavior. Relaxation and visualization techniques can be quite helpful in changing the patient's self-image to that of a healthy person, and these techniques can be initiated by, or at the direction of, a psychologist or similar professional.

The acupuncture treatment plan for smoking is almost identical to that for allergy with the addition of a staple (also called a *press pin*) in the inferior portion of the cavum conchae of each ear. This area is innervated by the cervical plexus. The area is first prepped with alcohol using a cotton-tipped applicator. After the alcohol dries, the press pin and its adhesive tape are placed using tweezers or pick-ups as shown in Figure 11.8a through Figure 11.8d. The staple is left in place for 2 weeks, although it is often necessary to replace it sooner because the adhesive tape does not hold up well in water, that is, the pool or the shower.

In the treatment session when the staple is placed, needles are also placed into the primary points. The patient is instructed to gently manipulate the staple periodically for additional stimulation, especially when experiencing the urge to smoke. The likelihood of smoking cessation is related to pain sensitivity level, with those at a higher degree requiring more treatment sessions: primary patients require one session; secondary, two; tertiary, three; and nonspecific, four. The needles in the primary points and the ear staples are placed in the first session and the primary points are needled every 2 or 3 days thereafter as necessary; in the latter sessions the ear staples are examined and replaced if they are not secure. The Paravertebral points (in the posterior cutaneous nerves of T2 through T5) are useful in smoking cessation when the patient is in the prone position.

For weight reduction, the only difference is the number and placement of the ear staples. Instead of being placed in the inferior cavum conchae area, two staples are placed higher, immediately above and below the conchum (Figure 11.9). This is the location of the auricular branch of the vagus nerve (see Figure 11.7d), and the needles are thought by the authors to interfere with digestive signals carried by the vagus. It is not necessary to needle the primary points in this setting.

Acupuncture can be a useful adjunct in treating other addictions, such as alcohol and drugs, by reducing pain and thus the need for self-medication. Also, acupuncture alone seems to reduce stress transiently, making the trauma of withdrawing from intoxicants less. Again, it would be naïve to expect acupuncture to do the job alone; it is only an adjunct to a comprehensive program in this difficult setting.

## 11.10 CONDITIONS AFFECTING THE SPECIAL SENSES

Generally speaking, acupuncture to treat conditions of the special senses is ineffective — with three limited exceptions. Restoration of the sense of smell can be achieved when loss of smell is associated with an allergic condition by treating the allergies as described earlier. Tinnitus and vertigo can sometimes be reduced when the origin of the problem is the middle ear by utilizing three sessions: the first is supine with all primary points and two in the front of each ear, the Temporomandibular (27) and the Auriculotemporal (U); the second is prone with the primary and Paravertebral points; and the third is sitting using primary and secondary points on the head, face, shoulders, and arms in addition to the two points anterior to each ear. Intraocular pressure can also be reduced with acupuncture, but only transiently; acupuncture should never be considered a definitive treatment for glaucoma.

## 11.11 OTHER CONDITIONS

Decreased tear secretion resulting in dry, irritated eyes has been reported to be relieved by acupuncture.[6] The report described the use of 10 points on the face and head; the authors' approach to this problem is to add the Lacrimal (102) point to the sinus allergy protocol.

Xerostomia, typically as a complication of radiation treatment for tumors of the head and neck, has been reported to respond to acupuncture.[7] The patients in this study were resistant to pilocarpine. To the basic protocol, the three points in the ear described earlier for smoking and weight reduction, along with the Superficial Radial (12) points, may be tried; other points that may alleviate this condition are Supraorbital (23), Infraorbital (19), Mental (50), Masseter (30), Temporomandibular (27), and nonspecific points found to be passive behind the inferior border of the mandible. The authors suspect that xerostomia in response to radiation may be more likely to develop in individuals who have a high pain sensitivity.

Depression is another adjunctive application for acupuncture; acupuncture patients frequently report requiring

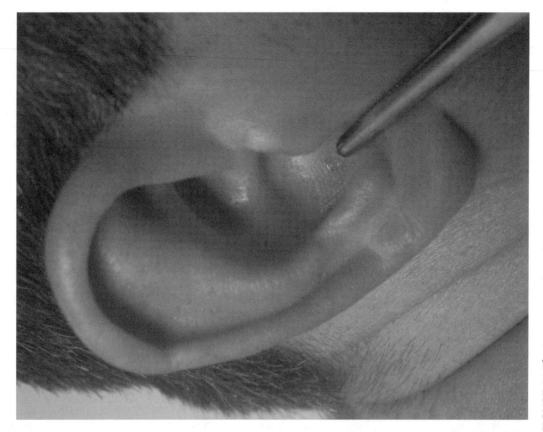

**FIGURE 11.8b** An ear press pin positioned for smoking cessation (continued): the press pin is positioned with tweezers.

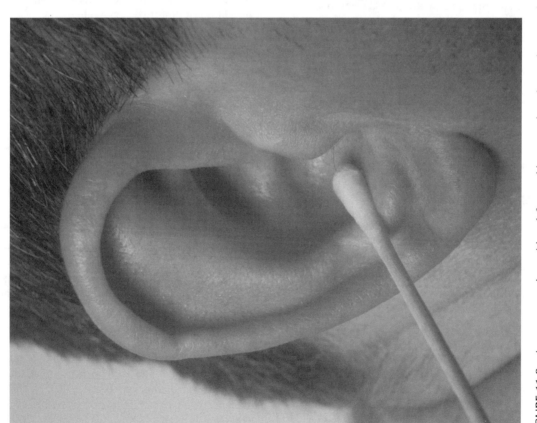

**FIGURE 11.8a** An ear press pin positioned for smoking cessation: the ear is prepped with an applicator moistened with alcohol.

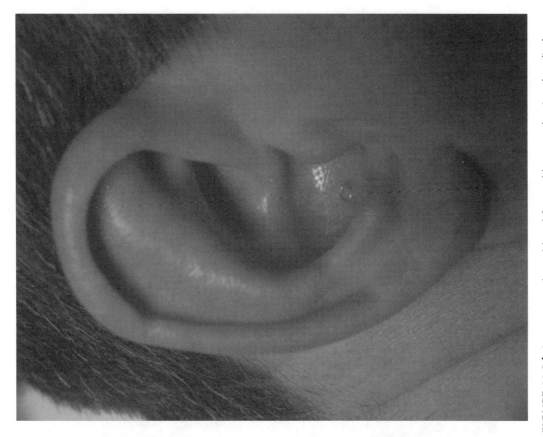

FIGURE 11.8d An ear press pin positioned for smoking cessation (continued): the press pin is firmly affixed and left in place with its adhesive backing for 2 weeks.

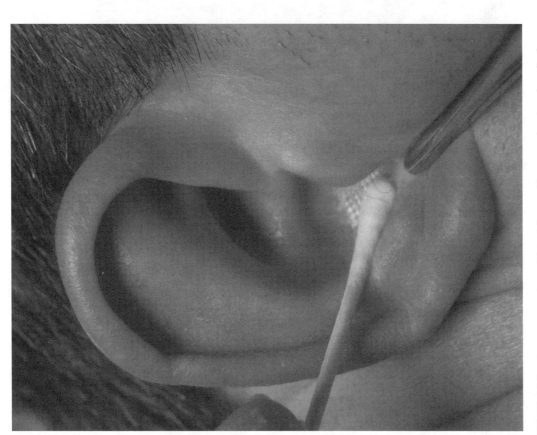

FIGURE 11.8c An ear press pin positioned for smoking cessation (continued): the press pin is pushed into the flesh of the ear with an applicator.

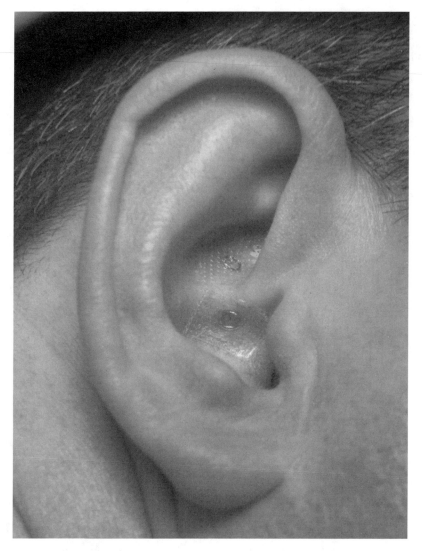

**FIGURE 11.9** Ear staples placed for weight loss.

lower dosages of antidepressant medication after under-going acupuncture. Of course, pain and depression often go hand in hand, and reduction in pain may reduce depression. Whether an independent mechanism exists is yet another area for further study. Anxiety may also be at least transiently affected, possibly by reduction in sympathetic tone after needling.

## 11.12  CONCLUSION

As the examples cited in this chapter show, acupuncture can be useful in treating many painful conditions of the head and face, especially in patients who are young, present early in the course of their disease, and have low pain sensitivity levels. Sinus allergy, a gratifying application of acupuncture that is most often successful, is independent of pain sensitivity. Addictions may be treated with acupuncture, but to be successful it is best to use acupuncture as a component of a multidisciplinary approach. Other

conditions in the face and head may respond to acupuncture, although much more research is needed in these areas.

## REFERENCES

1. Dung, H.C. Biostatistical profiles of individuals seeking acupuncture treatment in the United States. *Chin. Med. J.* 98:835, 1985.
2. Diamond, C. and Frew, J. *The Facial Nerve*. Oxford University Press, New York, 1979.
3. Graham, M.D. and House, W.F. *Disorders of the Facial Nerves: Anatomy, Diagnosis and Management*. Raven Press, New York, 1982.
4. Moldaver, J. and Conley, J. *The Facial Palsies, Their Physiopathy and Therapeutic Approaches*. Charles C Thomas, Springfield, IL, 1980.
5. Hauser, W.A. et al. Incidence and prognosis of Bell's palsy in the population of Rochester, Minnesota. *Mayo Clin. Proc.* 46:258, 1971.

6. Nepp, J. et al. Dry eye treatment with acupuncture. In *Lacrimal Gland, Tear Film, and Dry Eye Syndromes 2*, Sullivan, D.A. et al., Eds., Plenum Press, New York, 1998.

7. Johnstone, P.A.S. et al. Acupuncture for pilocarpine-resistant xerostomia following radiotherapy for head and neck malignancies. *Int. J. Radiol. Oncol. Biol. Phys.* 50:353, 2001.

# 12 Conditions of the Neck, Shoulders, and Upper Extremities

## CONTENTS

## 12.1 OVERVIEW

When a young, fair-skinned female presents to the clinic complaining of neck pain, investigation usually uncovers a history of dysmenorrhea and relatively low blood pressure. These patients are also likely to have long menstrual periods with excessive blood loss and, as a result of years of dysmenorrhea, relatively high pain sensitivities. As a rule of thumb, every 5 years of dysmenorrhea adds one degree to pain sensitivity. (As an example, a 43-year-old female who started having painful menses at age 13 would have a 30-year history of dysmenorrhea and, absent any other sources of pain, would be expected to have a sensitivity of 30/5 = 6.) Pain in the neck and shoulder is a very common indication for acupuncture; the often causative dysmenorrhea can and should be treated as well, as described in the next chapter. Because the neck, shoulder, and upper extremities are innervated by the cervical plexus and the brachial plexus, which have some interconnections at the level of the upper brachial plexus, they are considered together.

## 12.2 ACUPUNCTURE AND NEUROANATOMY OF THE NECK AND SHOULDERS

The cervical nerve plexus (CNP) is formed by the interconnecting branches of the ventral primary rami of the first four cervical spinal nerves and contains cutaneous and muscular branches. The muscular branch (the ansa cervicalis) is not clinically significant because it supplies the fairly minor infrahyoid muscles (the sternohyoid, sternothyroid, thyrohyoid, and omohyoid). The CNP has four cutaneous branches with 11 acupoints among them. Acupoints formed by CNP have been previously reported.[1] The cutaneous branches emerge through the muscle layer behind the midpoint of the posterior border of the sternocleidomastoid muscle that runs from the mastoid process to the sternal end of the clavicle and the manubrium. At this midpoint, easily estimated by placing a thumb on the sternoclavicular joint and forefinger on the mastoid process, a rather deep acupoint, the Cervical Plexus (28), marks the emergence and division of the nerve into the four branches: the great auricular, lesser occipital, transverse cervical, and supraclavicular.

Each of the branches has associated acupoints (see Figure 12.1a and Figure 12.1b). The greater auricular nerve crosses the sternocleidomastoid muscle obliquely to course toward the ear, where it emerges from the investing fascia just behind the lowest point of the earlobe, forming the important Great Auricular (2) acupoint. The lesser occipital nerve, a cutaneous nerve containing fibers from the first two cervical spinal nerves, ascends from the cervical plexus, generally without branching, along the posterior border of the sternocleidomastoid muscle. It pierces the cervical investing fascia near the intermuscular gap between the insertions of the sternocleidomastoid and the trapezius on the occipital bone. Here, the Lesser Occipital (34) acupoint is formed as the nerve branches to innervate the skin behind the ear. The greater auricular and lesser occipital nerves illustrate that larger nerve size predisposes to the early development of acupoints because the two are similar except that the greater auricular is larger and its acupoint becomes passive earlier in the progression of pain sensitivity.

The transverse cervical nerve courses anteriorly, horizontally across the sternocleidomastoid, where it divides into three bundles at the anterior border of the muscle before piercing the deep fascia. These branches innervate the skin of the anterior triangle of the neck and form several acupoints in a small cluster where they become cutaneous; these points are collectively identified as the Transverse Cervical (53) acupoints. The supraclavicular nerve, like the transverse cervical, divides into several branches before piercing the deep fascia to become superficial. These branches course to the clavicle, forming three pairs of acupoints: the Medial Supraclavicular (85); the Intermediate Supraclavicular (80); and the Lateral Supraclavicular (86). Each branch can form two acupoints — one on the superior border of the clavicle and the other on the inferior border — and these point pairs are named collectively.

Two other cutaneous nerves arising from the posterior primary rami of the cervical spinal nerves contribute important acupoints: the greater occipital nerve with its Greater Occipital (7) acupoint and the third occipital with its Third Occipital (U) acupoint. The greater occipital nerve emerges between the posterior arch of the atlas and the lamina of the axis immediately below the obliquus capitis inferior muscle; it becomes subcutaneous in the concavity of the suboccipital triangle area, piercing the deep fascia immediately lateral to the insertion of the trapezius muscle on the superior occipital nuchal line. The greater occipital acupoint is located between the insertions of trapezius and sternocleidomastoid muscles. It is a very important point used in almost all patients, especially those with headache and neck pain. The Third Occipital point is 2 to 3 cm inferolateral to the Greater Occipital point.

It should be pointed out that other investigators[2] in the field of algology have suggested that trigger or motor points in the anterior cervical triangle are formed on the scalene muscles. However, we are somewhat skeptical because the scalene muscles are very deep in the neck. It is questionable whether tenderness in these muscles can be palpated from the skin surface. Also, because of the many huge nerve trunks and large vessels nearby, it would be risky to place needles so deep.

The spinal accessory (XI) nerve and its interconnecting branches from the second and third cervical spinal nerves have afferent and efferent branches to two muscles: the sternocleidomastoid and trapezius (see Figure 12.1a and Figure 12.1b). Only the trapezius branch is clinically significant because the sternocleidomastoid neuromuscular attachments rarely become tender while those of the trapezius may become so reactive as to form a nodule that feels like a rock when pierced by a needle. The Spinal Accessory-I (3) acupoint is almost always tender in chronic pain sufferers, and those with neck and shoulder pain may have several tender acupoints over the shoulder bridge in the middle area of the muscle.

The skin and musculature of the upper extremities, including the shoulder, are innervated by the brachial plexus, with the exception of a small area of skin on the shoulder. The upper extremity is generally divided into the shoulder, arm (brachium), forearm (antebrachium), wrist (carpus), and hand (manus). The shoulder consists of the shoulder girdle (the clavicle and scapula) and the muscles attached to it. The arm is formed by the humerus and the muscles surrounding it, including muscles from anterior and posterior surfaces of the thorax. Muscles attached to the shoulder and brachium, such as the rhomboids, pectoralis, supraspinatus, and infraspinatus, are innervated by branches of the brachial plexus. The forearm has two bones: the radius and ulna; more than 20 muscles attach to these two bones. The wrist refers to eight small bones in the carpal region and the hand is made of the metacarpal bones, phalanges, and muscles in the palm.

All of these structures result from outgrowth of a single limb bud during embryological development; this bud is followed by the ventral primary rami of spinal nerves from C4 to T1. These rami form three trunks that then divide into anterior (or "preaxial") and posterior (or "postaxial") divisions to innervate, respectively, the anterior and posterior aspects of the upper thorax and upper extremity. The anterior division eventually forms the lateral and medial pectoral nerves, musculocutaneous nerve, median nerve, and ulnar nerve to innervate the preaxial musculatures, including the two pectoral muscles in the anterior thoracic region, muscles of the anterior compartment in the brachium, muscles in the medial compartment of the antebrachium, and intrinsic muscles in the palms of the hands.

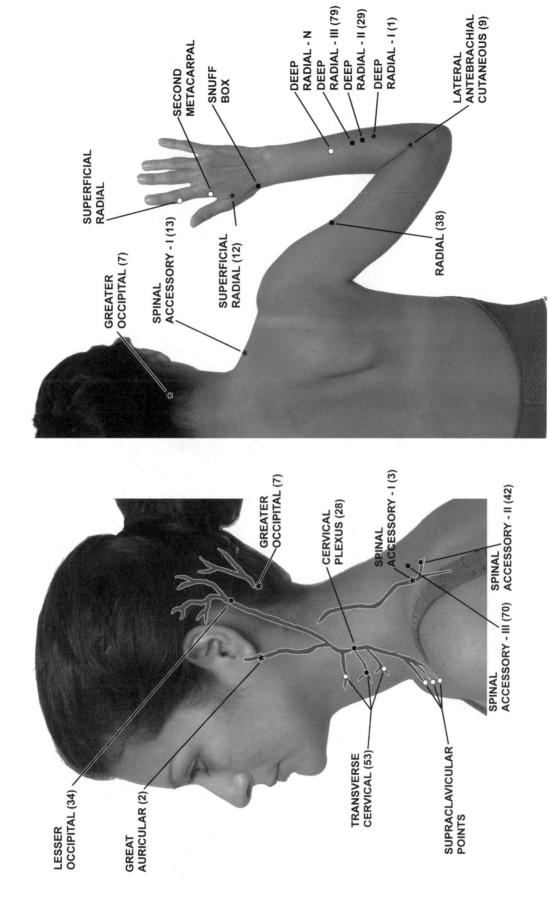

**FIGURE 12.1b** Some acupoints of the neck and shoulder: posterolateral view.

**FIGURE 12.1a** Some acupoints of the neck and shoulder: lateral view.

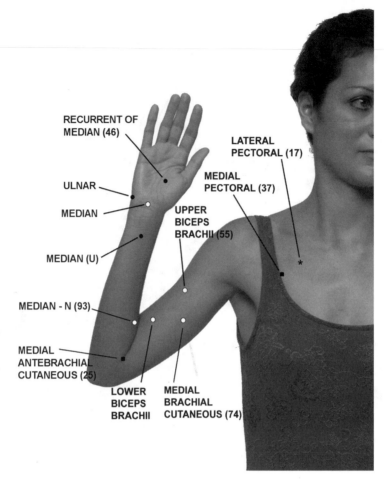

**FIGURE 12.2a** Acupoints arising from the brachial plexus: anterior view.

Cutaneous nerves originating from the anterior division include the medial brachial cutaneous, medial antebrachial cutaneous, and lateral antebrachial cutaneous nerves. The posterior division forms the dorsal scapular, suprascapular, axillary, and radial nerves to innervate the postaxial musculatures including the levator scapulae, rhomboid major and minor, supraspinatus and infraspinatus in the shoulder and posterior thoracic regions, muscles in the posterior compartment of the brachium, and muscles in the lateral compartment of the antebrachium. No muscles are in the dorsal aspects of the hands. Cutaneous nerves from the posterior division include the posterior brachial cutaneous, posterior antebrachial cutaneous, and superficial radial nerves. All of the acupoints in the upper extremities and shoulder girdle originate from these nerves (see Figure 12.2a through Figure 12.2c).

Acupoints from the anterior division include:

- Lateral Pectoral (17) in the middle of the pectoralis major muscle
- Medial Pectoral (37) 3 to 4 cm inferior and lateral to the Lateral Pectoral acupoint

- Upper Biceps Brachii (55), which is the upper neuromuscular attachment of the musculocutaneous nerve to the biceps muscle (a lower attachment is clinically insignificant)
- Lateral Antebrachial Cutaneous (9) formed by the lateral antebrachial cutaneous nerve that is the distal portion of the musculocutaneous nerve at the lateral border of the cubital fossa
- Medial Brachial Cutaneous (74) from the similarly named nerve and located on the medial surface of the brachium midway between the axillary pit and medial epicondyle of the humerus
- Medial Antebrachial Cutaneous (25) from the similarly named nerve, accompanied by the basilic vein, at the location where the nerve pierces the deep fascia slightly anterior to the medial epicondyle at the elbow on the medial end of the cubital fossa
- Median (U) formed by the median nerve where it emerges from under the palmaris longus muscle (which it innervates, along with other long flexor muscles of the forearm)

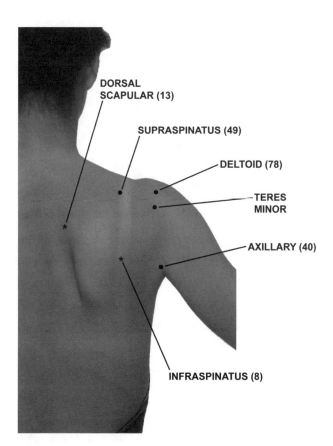

**FIGURE 12.2b** Acupoints arising from the brachial plexus: posterior view of shoulder.

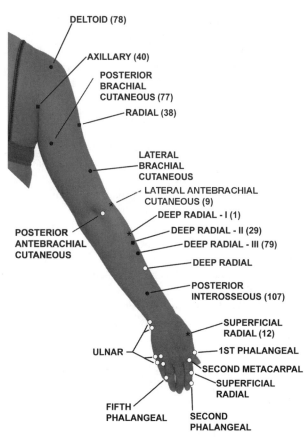

**FIGURE 12.2c** Acupoints arising from the brachial plexus: posterior view of upper extremity.

- Recurrent of Median (46) formed by the recurrent branch of the median nerve as it loops back through the palm to innervate the muscles of the thenar eminence
- Nonspecific points along the ulnar nerve on the ulnar side of the wrist and hand

Nerves and musculature of the anterior and posterior divisions of the brachial plexus exist in a rough balance, not surprising given that muscle actions in one direction (e.g., flexion) need to be balanced by actions in the opposite direction (e.g., extension). The eight named acupoints of the posterior division are

1. The Dorsal Scapular (13) derives from the dorsal scapular nerve, which innervates the levator scapulae, rhomboid major, and rhomboid minor muscles, at the neuromuscular attachment of the nerve with the rhomboid minor along the medial border of the scapula. This point becomes painful so often that it has not escaped the notice of clinical scientists such as Calabro,[3] Campbell,[4] Sheon et al.,[5] and Travell and Simons.[2] Calabro noted that patients with fibro-

myalgia pain have a 28% chance of having tenderness at this point.

2,3. The Infraspinatus (8) and Supraspinatus (49) acupoints are neuromuscular attachments of the suprascapular nerve to the infraspinatus and supraspinatus muscles respectively. The neuromuscular attachment on the supraspinatus muscle is established after the nerve passes through the suprascapular foramen under the suprascapular ligament on the superior border of the scapula. The supraspinatus is a round muscle with a thick mass in the supraspinatus fossa. The nerve reaches the muscle mass from underneath so that the neuromuscular attachment is deeply located. In contrast to the branch that enters the infraspinatus muscle, the point under the supraspinatus is harder to palpate and less likely to be tender. After supplying the muscular branch to the supraspinatus, the suprascapular nerve curves around the scapular notch to form a neuromuscular attachment with the infraspinatus, a broad muscle with a thin mass, at the center of the infraspinatus fossa. The infraspinatus acupoint always becomes tender before the supraspinatus, reflecting the fact that, although the nerve is more or less the same size at the two points, it is more superficial at its attachment to the infraspinatus muscle.

4. The Axillary (40) acupoint in the posterior axillary fold is considered to be in the upper extremity. The axillary nerve passes through the quadrangular space to reach the back of the shoulder joint and winds around the surgical neck of the humerus to innervate the teres minor and the deltoid muscles. Branches of the axillary nerve entering the teres minor and the deltoid can also form acupoints at their neuromuscular attachments, for example, the Deltoid (78).

5. The Posterior Brachial Cutaneous (77) acupoint is a cutaneous point at which the posterior brachial cutaneous nerve, a branch of the radial nerve, pierces the deep fascia. After leaving the axillary region, the radial nerve runs downward, backward, and laterally between the long and medial heads of the triceps to enter the radial groove of the humerus. The trunk of the radial nerve can be palpated at the location where it lies in the groove immediately below the insertion of the deltoid muscle. At this location, the radial nerve gives off the posterior antebrachial cutaneous nerve supplying the skin of the posterior surface of the forearm, and it is at this point of bifurcation that the Radial (38) acupoint is found.

6. The Radial acupoint is fairly insignificant because of its depth in the muscle mass. The radial nerve then penetrates the lateral intermuscular septum of the brachium to enter the anterior compartment of the arm, where it divides into two terminal branches: the deep and superficial radial nerves.

7. The deep radial nerve forms the Deep Radial-I (1) acupoint, the most important in the body because it is the first in the sequence of acupoint progression to become tender, most likely because of its size and depth, bifurcations, and its association with the radial artery and vein, and also because it is a nerve forming neuromuscular attachments. Because of the rotation of the forearm during embryologic development, the flexor compartment that is initially located anteriorly migrates to the ulnar or medial side, while the extensor compartment becomes laterally located at the radial side. The deep radial nerve enters the lateral or extensor compartment of the forearm to supply the extensor muscles of the wrist and fingers. The superficial radial nerve emerges under the cover of the brachioradialis muscle at the distal portion of the radius, where acupoints are likely to form over the surface overlying the nerve in

patients suffering from superficial radial nerve neuropathy or neuralgia, often caused by direct injury to the nerve such as a blow to the radius bone near the wrist. Proximal to the wrist, the nerve running along the surface of the radius is still covered by the deep fascia and has no branches. As it continues distally beyond the radius, the nerve begins to branch in the anatomic snuffbox and on the web between the thumb and index finger. The snuffbox is immediately distal to the styloid process of the radius, and at this location an acupoint can be formed.

8. The most important acupoint of the superficial radial nerve is exactly in the middle of the web between the thumb and index finger — the Superficial Radial (12) point. The posterior antebrachial nerve, a cutaneous nerve that pierces the brachial (deep) fascia between the lateral epicondyle of the humerus and the olecranon of the radius above the elbow, may form a minor acupoint sometimes associated with lateral epicondylitis (tennis elbow).

The other acupoints in the upper extremity are not associated with specific nerve elements. These include the biceps tendon between the greater and lesser tubercles of the humerus; the lateral epicondyle, the attachment point for many of the long flexor muscles of the forearm; the medial epicondyle, the attachment point for forearm extensor muscles; the so-called basal joint, or carpometacarpal joint, at the base of the thumb; and the proximal interphalangeal and distal interphalangeal joints of the fingers.

## 12.3 ACUPUNCTURE APPLIED TO CONDITIONS OF THE NECK, SHOULDER, AND UPPER EXTREMITY

A number of painful conditions in the neck, shoulders, and upper extremity, such as cervical strain or sprain, respond quite well to acupuncture, depending on pain sensitivity level; others, such as arthritis, respond poorly. One extremely common presentation is so noteworthy as to deserve special mention. Patients will frequently describe their neck and shoulder pain as experienced in three areas corresponding exactly to three acupoints: the Greater Occipital (7), Spinal Accessory-I (3), and Dorsal Scapular (13). Patients will draw out the location of the pain as shown in Figure 12.3.

This pain can be seen to be associated with the second, third, and fourth spinal nerves. The greater occipital nerve is derived from the posterior primary ramus of C2; afferent or sensory fibers that enter the trapezius by way of the spinal accessory nerve are derived from C2 and C3; and the dorsal scapular nerve is a branch of the brachial plexus

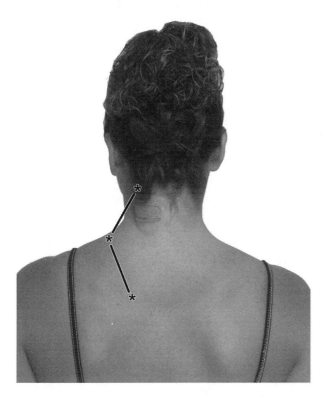

**FIGURE 12.3** Patients with neck and shoulder pain will often draw out the locations of these three acupoints in describing their pain. Shown on the model's left side, the three points are, from superior to inferior: the Greater Occipital (7); Spinal Accessory-I (3); and Dorsal Scapular (13). These are all primary points.

derived from the anterior primary ramus of C4. (The exact derivation of the spinal accessory nerve has been simplified because its relationship to the vagus nerve is controversial and unnecessarily complex for the purposes of this text.) These interconnections among the three spinal nerves are the most likely explanation of this frequent pain distribution, especially common in slender females between 35 and 45 years old who have relatively low blood pressure and dysmenorrhea. When treating such patients, the physician should be sure to place at least one needle in each of the three points; two or three needles in each point may be indicated.

### 12.3.1 Muscle Pain in the Neck and Shoulders

Pain in the neck and shoulders caused by acute or chronic muscular strain or sprain goes by a number of names, such as occipital headache, tension headache, and whiplash. These conditions are first associated with tenderness of the primary Greater Occipital acupoint. As they progress, the secondary Lesser Occipital (34) and Third Occipital (U)* points become tender and, as the number

---

\* This acupoint, the posterior cutaneous nerve of the posterior primary ramus of C3, is located two centimeters inferior to the Greater Occipital (7) acupoint.

of tender points increases, the pain becomes more difficult to manage. Most of these patients, however, have pain sensitivities of six or less and these conditions are generally responsive to acupuncture. Many of these seem to be related to hormonal fluctuations, as is the case with Lisa, a 31-year-old housewife.

Lisa came to the clinic complaining of occipital headache and stating that it was worse right before ovulation. When asked to localize her headache, she placed her finger on the Greater Occipital acupoint. She was found to have a pain sensitivity of four degrees, with only a few secondary points in the passive phase. She was having a headache when she presented, a few days before her expected ovulation. For her first session, she was treated in the supine position with needles only in the primary points. For the second, she was treated in the prone position with needles in the dorsal primary points. She was told to wait a few days for ovulation to occur before coming for a third visit. At the third visit, she had ovulated without having any further headache. At that time she was placed in the sitting position, and all the primary and secondary points in her head and neck were needled. She was told to return in 4 weeks if her headache recurred, but she did not come back and it was felt that her problem had resolved.

Patients who present at five degrees or more are treated initially as described previously, additionally receiving needles in the Lesser Occipital and Third Occipital points at each visit. For difficult headaches, increasing numbers of needles are employed to try to obtain a response. If particular muscles such as the trapezius, splenius capitus, and sternocleidomastoid show tender points, four to six needles can be added in the tender areas.

Whiplash, or cervical sprain/strain, is another condition distinguished from occipital headache in that it has a discrete onset, usually related to a vehicular accident. It should be noted that financial factors, such as ongoing litigation, may make treatment difficult. Although the term *whiplash* can be used to describe severe injuries resulting in vertebral fractures and damage to spinal nerves, it is most often applied to pure soft tissue injury. The third through seventh cervical spinal nerve distribution is most often affected; the pain can be localized to a single nerve's distribution or generalized as more spinal nerves are affected. It is uncertain whether a nerve is primarily affected by stretching or if it is reactive to reduced blood supply and increasing release of toxins from muscle spasm and damage. With more extensive tissue injury, these cases can be difficult to manage.

One example is Shari, a freshman medical student who wore a cervical collar to the acupuncture clinic after she was in a motor vehicle accident (MVA). As final examinations approached, she was anxious to be rid of the pain. She was found to have no tender acupoints outside the cervical area. The Lesser Occipital, Greater Occipital, Greater Auricular, Third Occipital, Cervical Plexus, Spinal

Accessory-I, Dorsal Scapular, and Infraspinatus points were tender. Because of her low sensitivity and youth, it was anticipated that she would be easy to treat. Her pain totally resolved with one treatment, administered while she was in the sitting position, with needles placed only at the eight points on each side that were passive.

Another example is Kuang-Hua, a 29-year-old Taiwanese Air Force captain. He was estimated to have a pain sensitivity of four but, because he was seen shortly after the MVA that caused his injury, he was easily treated, even though on initial presentation he was in such pain that he was unable to turn his head to either side and had difficulty sleeping. His first session was administered in the supine position, with the ventral primary points plus the Lesser Occipital (34), Third Occipital (U), Biceps Tendon (U), Cervical Plexus (28), and Spinal Accessory-II (42) points needled. On his second visit 2 days later, the pain was significantly reduced, and he was needled in the prone position with the primary points and the same additional points used as in the first visit. The next day a cold front arrived, and on the third visit he noted a flare-up of pain that he attributed to the cold; he was again having difficulty turning his head from side to side. At that visit, he was treated in the sitting position and all primary, secondary, and a few tertiary points in the neck, shoulder, and upper extremities were needled. On his fourth visit, he related that his pain was 80% resolved. He had a total of six sessions, the last three repeating the first three. On the last visit, the patient was asymptomatic.

In contrast to these two successes, patients with high sensitivities and long-standing conditions are difficult to manage. One example is Sylvia, a 70-year-old female who had injured her neck in an MVA 30 years previously. She had a sensitivity of nine degrees and was felt to have palpable knots in her trapezius, a sign of long-standing muscle tension. She had a total of 22 treatments with temporary reductions of symptoms followed by inevitable recurrences, a common scenario for high-degree sufferers.

Along with high pain sensitivity and a long-standing condition, one negative prognostic indicator for muscular neck pain is tenderness in several terminal branches of the transverse cervical and supraclavicular nerves. Finally, the authors have anecdotal evidence to suggest that high-sensitivity patients may be likely to have more neck pain after MVAs, but this requires scientific investigation before any conclusions are reached.

### 12.3.2 Arthritic Pain and Degenerative Disk Disease

Osteoarthritic pain in the neck does not usually respond well to acupuncture for a couple of reasons. It is usually long-standing, suggesting a high pain sensitivity level, by the time acupuncture treatment is sought. Also, a structural change, such as spurring and facet joint degeneration, has

usually taken place in the arthritic neck, and acupuncture is not going to affect structure. The same can more or less be said for degenerative intervertebral disk disease: the painful condition is typically long-standing, so acupuncture is not going to improve the structure of desiccated disks. Nevertheless, patients often have an improvement in subjective pain perception, at least temporarily, and increased mobility after acupuncture treatments.

One positive example is Jean, a 63-year-old retiree, who had been diagnosed with arthritis in the fourth, fifth, and sixth cervical vertebrae and significant degenerative disk disease. She had pain and very limited motion in her neck, with a pain sensitivity of seven. She obtained substantial relief with increased mobility and decreased pain after 12 treatment sessions over a 2-month period. She returned to clinic 12 years later because she had sustained additional injury in a skiing accident. She said that since her earlier course of treatment, her severe pain had resolved with just occasional mild aching. Her pain from her reinjury resolved after only two treatments. Jean is somewhat atypical in that many patients do not have such impressive results. It may be that her pain was wrongly attributed to her arthritis and disk disease when she was first diagnosed.

### 12.3.3 Post-Herpetic Pain in the Neck

Pain in the neck can be a sequela of herpes zoster, discussed in some detail in the previous chapter. One case involving at least four dermatomes was effectively managed with acupuncture using the same approach previously described.

### 12.3.4 Pain Radiating from the Neck to the Upper Extremity

Pain radiating down the radial or the ulnar side of the arm from the neck is fairly common. Occasionally the pain does not follow a dermatomal distribution but affects the entire limb. The causes are often difficult to ascertain and can include herniated cervical disk, foraminal stenosis, or injury to a peripheral nerve at any point along its length. Pinched or stretched nerves can cause pain, numbness, and paresthesias. The mechanical problems must be addressed because even if acupuncture temporarily relieves the pain, it will recur. Sometimes the mechanical problems can be alleviated but the pain remains; an example is a carpal tunnel syndrome patient who continues to have pain after the median nerve is surgically decompressed. These cases can be extraordinarily complex and the diagnosis elusive, even after MRIs and nerve conduction testing. Often these patients have multiple complaints, as the next example shows.

Charles G. was a 43-year-old marine engine repairman when he first came to the clinic complaining of neck pain. He had seen seven different doctors, one of whom had written:

His primary complaint is severe neck pain which radiates into the left shoulder and arm. He has numbness and tingling in the left upper extremity, but cannot localize the paresthesias. He has weakness in the left upper extremity, but is limited by pain. He wakes at night with pain and numbness in his hand and arm. He also describes lower back pain, but this symptom is improving. He describes vascular headache, which begins in the posterior occipital head regions. He attributes his symptoms to an injury suffered at work.... He was driving his vehicle looking for a child lost at work, and he was rear-ended. He was wearing his seatbelt, and suffered a flexion–extension injury. He may have struck his head, but he cannot remember. He did not lose consciousness, but his memory was impaired for 20 minutes after the accident....

Charles G. had ultimately been found to be at maximum medical improvement (MMI) and rated at a 38% disability.* He gradually returned to work with these restrictions: "no work that would require the use of his left hand; no prolonged standing or sitting; no lifting, pulling, tearing; no prolonged driving or sitting in a vehicle; and time allowed to continue physical therapy." Imaging revealed disc degeneration with misalignment of the posterior aspect of the C5–C6 vertebral bodies, and the problem list from his physician had been generated as follows: "(1) neuropathy distal to left elbow; (2) neuropathy of the right hand; (3) loss of fine movement in hands — cannot write well; (4) severe and constant pain in the left neck and left arm; (5) right hip pain; and (6) low back pain."

Despite these multiple injuries, his pain sensitivity was only two, and it was felt that he could benefit from acupuncture. The length of time from his injury to presentation for acupuncture treatment (6 years) was a negative prognostic factor, but he had previously been healthy and athletic, a positive factor. His first treatment was while he was in the prone position with primary points needled. On his second visit, he complained of significant pain in his left shoulder, medial side of his left elbow, and palmar side of his left hand. He was placed in the supine position and needles were placed in all primary acupoints — plus four along the tendon of the left biceps brachii in the bicipital groove, four over the medial epicondyle of the left humerus, and two in points along the median nerve in the left distal forearm, including the Median (U), and the Recurrent of Median (46). On his third visit, his affect was much improved and he said he had experienced several pain-free hours. On that visit, he was placed in the sitting position and treated with needles in the primary points and in the same left hand, arm, and shoulder points used in the second visit. After that visit, he did not require any further treatment.

---

* This number seems high. The case occurred in 1994 in Texas and was probably rated in accordance with an early edition of the *AMA Guides*, the authoritative source of rating methodology. Later editions have become more restrictive.

His favorable outcome can be related to his low sensitivity and his previously healthy condition.

This example also illustrates another point. Needles are generally placed in the area where the patient perceives symptoms and along the nerve trunks leading to that area, as in this case in which needles were placed along the median nerve leading to the hand as well as in the hand itself. If the diagnosis is unclear, the patient will often benefit by simply placing needles in areas where the patient perceives pain, numbness, and tingling, and in all the passive acupoints in the area.

One example of this latter point is Charles R., a 51-year-old salesman who complained of approximately 15 years of pain in his right shoulder; the pain began at the shoulder and ran down to the arm, forearm, and hand along the route of the radial, deep radial, and superficial radial nerves. Charles had undergone neck surgery in 1966 when he was 21 years old. The surgery completely relieved his pain for about a decade; then it began to return. This initial success probably reflected low pain sensitivity at the time of surgery because his sensitivity at the time of presenting for acupuncture was a mere three degrees.

His first session took place when he was in the prone position, with needles placed in the primary points along with two needles placed 2 and 5 cm inferior to the dorsal scapular point along the medial scapular border. On his second visit, he related that his pain was substantially reduced and that his sleep had improved. At that visit he was placed in the supine position for needles to be placed in the primary points and four additional points along the tendon of the right biceps brachii muscle in the intertubercular sulcus or bicipital groove. The biceps tendon is almost always tender in patients with shoulder pain. When Charles presented for his third visit, the pain was practically gone; he was placed in a sitting position and special emphasis was placed on primary and secondary points in the right shoulder and arm.

After that, we lost contact with him for nearly a decade; then he returned to say that he had been pain free the entire time until, a few weeks before, his right shoulder and neck began to hurt again, so much so that he would wake up three times a night. He saw his private physician and an MRI was done that showed arthritic changes in the cervical spine; surgery was again recommended but instead he came for three more acupuncture treatments similar to his previous ones. We think the relapse was due to his having had cervical surgery before coming for acupuncture treatments; prior surgery is one variable that often confounds the assessment techniques presented in this text and almost always worsens the prognosis.

### 12.3.5 Pain in the Shoulder Joint

The shoulder joint is the direct or indirect articulation formed among the lateral end of the clavicle, the coracoid process, the acromion, the glenoid cavity of the scapula, and the head of the humerus. Pain in this joint is quite common; it is a complaint of about 10% of our patients. Most authorities consider rotator cuff pathology to be the major cause of shoulder pain,[6–8] but we consider that the role of the richly innervated biceps tendon in the intertubercular groove is underestimated. In our experience, shoulder pain can be managed fairly well with acupuncture, suggesting that a structural component to these patients' pain is lacking.

Patients with shoulder pain will almost always have one or more acupoints in the passive phase along the biceps tendon. Pain in the shoulder has a tendency to spread posterolaterally around the acromion to the area of the deltoid muscle; the further the pain spreads in this direction the more difficult it will be to manage. This movement of the pain as indicated by passive acupoints over the acromion and deltoid suggests involvement of the rotator cuff, which consists of the tendons of four muscles (teres minor; infraspinatus; supraspinatus; and subscapularis) that nearly encircle the humeral head. When the Acromioclavicular (52) and then the Deltoid (78) acupoints become passive, pain in such a condition will be progressively difficult to manage with acupuncture alone.

Elmer, age 61, is a typical example. He described his problem as a "pinched nerve" in his left shoulder with pain in the joint that had been bothering him for about 5 years. He had been otherwise healthy (except for a low back problem kept at bay with a home exercise program), could not identify any precipitating injury, and had had no surgeries. Generally, patients who can manage their back pain with exercise have a relatively low pain sensitivity; Elmer's was estimated at four degrees. He had tried a chiropractor for adjustments and his physician had given him pain medicine and muscle relaxants, but nothing seemed to provide lasting relief. He pointed to the Greater Occipital (7) point as the origin of his pain and indicated that the pain spread inferiorly to the Spinal Accessory-I (3) and further to the Dorsal Scapular (13). He perceived pain also within the shoulder joint itself. He had a lifelong history of relatively low blood pressure in the 110/70 range; low blood pressure is fairly common among patients of middle age presenting with neck and shoulder pain. The only tender points in his shoulder other than the three primary points already mentioned were along the biceps tendon (see Figure 12.4). His range of motion was normal, but he complained of slight pain along the biceps tendon with full extension and abduction of the shoulder joint.

The pain in Elmer's shoulder took only two acupuncture treatments to eliminate. The first was given to him while he was in the sitting position because of the rather intense pain along the axis from the greater occipital inferolaterally to the shoulder joint and inferiorly to the dorsal scapular acupoint. The patient's sitting upright is the most convenient position for placing needles in this

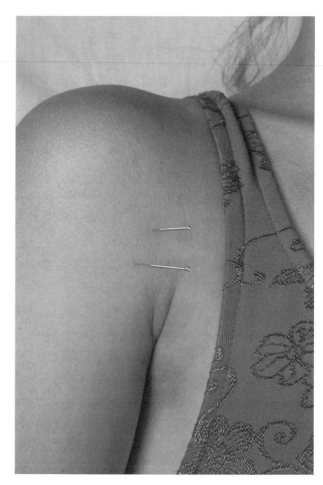

**FIGURE 12.4** Needle locations for treating pain along the biceps brachii tendon at the shoulder.

region, but it is fairly likely to cause syncope, especially in a new patient on his or her first visit. In addition to the primary points, a total of six needles were added in a row along each of Elmer's biceps tendons, left and right. When he came for his second treatment 2 days later, Elmer stated that his pain had eased and that he had slept well the past two nights. He was then placed in the supine position and needles were placed in all the accessible primary points and into both biceps tendons as before.

Another patient, Jane, who injured her shoulder working out with weights, represents a treatment failure after five sessions of acupuncture. She had only three degrees of sensitivity and her previous X-rays had been negative. The authors believe the treatment failed because the patient had been taking Demerol® and Percodan® before, during, and after her acupuncture treatments. We have observed that the influence of these drugs makes acupuncture relatively ineffective.

Although other treatment failures have occurred because of rotator cuff tears, calcium deposits, and high degrees of pain sensitivity, pain in the shoulder is usually easy to manage with acupuncture.

## 12.3.6 Pain in the Arm (Brachium)

Pain in the brachium (i.e., between the surgical neck and the supracondylar ridge of the humerus) is rare — a fact that probably reflects the paucity of acupoints in the region. The pain may be localized, in which case the treatment is to place a number of needles nonspecifically in the local area, or generalized, as in one case of post-herpetic pain involving the entire arm. In the latter case, needles should be placed in all the detectable tender points around the margins of the eruption.

## 12.3.7 Pain in the Elbow

The elbow is the joint between the distal end of the humerus and the proximal ends of the radius and ulna. Bony elements in the joint include the lateral and medial epicondyles, capitulum and trochlea of the humerus, the head of the radius, and the head and olecranon of the ulna. Most pain in the elbow originates from the lateral ("tennis elbow") and medial ("backhand tennis elbow" or "golf elbow") epicondyles or, more precisely, from the muscular attachments to the epicondyles.

Lateral epicondylitis is inflammation at the tendinous origin of the extensor muscles, such as the extensors carpi radialis longus and brevis in the forearm. Patients with this condition generally have good results with acupuncture, although patients with bilateral pain are typically more difficult to manage.

Richard, a right-handed retiree who spent much of his spare time playing tennis, complained of pain in the *left* elbow over the lateral epicondyle. His pain sensitivity was estimated at five degrees. On his first visit he was placed in the supine position; needles were placed in the primary points, six additional needles were inserted over the origins of the extensor muscles covering lateral epicondyle of the left humerus, and three additional needles were placed over the right lateral epicondyle, where tender points could be detected despite the absence of pain. On the second visit, the pain was not much reduced, and he was placed in the prone position and treated in the primary points and the elbow points as on his first visit. On the third visit, his pain was substantially reduced; he was placed in the sitting position and needles were placed in all the primary and secondary points in both upper limbs and points over the lateral epicondyles as before.

Richard was asked to wait for 5 days and then return for one or two more treatments if the pain in the elbow persisted. He did return for a fourth treatment because a slight residual pain could still be perceived, particularly when the left arm was forcefully swung. The second treatment was repeated. His fifth and last treatment 5 days later was identical to that of the first visit. He was not seen for 6 years; he then came to the clinic accompanying another patient and related that his left elbow had not bothered him since his last treatment.

Richard's case was fairly typical: tennis elbow patients present frequently, approximately one case every 2 to 3 weeks in Dung's clinic. Most will experience relief in six or fewer visits, the latter visits separated from the first three by a lapse of about a week. They are treated in the supine, prone, and sitting positions in sequence. An advantage to having patients in the sitting position is that more points in the elbow area are accessible; the disadvantage is a higher likelihood for the patients to develop syncope. The sitting position is to be avoided for the first and second acupuncture treatments for all new patients as much as possible; although syncope is easy to manage, it is distressing for the patient, especially one who has not experienced acupuncture before.

One point to be emphasized with patients with epicondylitis sustained as a result of sports is the importance of resting the affected part during the period of acupuncture treatments and for some time thereafter. Otherwise, the pain may well recur. Some patients continue to have recurrences of epicondylitis caused by continued sports activities.

In the authors' experience, medial epicondylitis is less frequently encountered than lateral epicondylitis — a ratio of about 1:20. The treatment principles are the same, except that needles are placed medially rather than laterally. Pain over the medial epicondyle is often attributed to ulnar nerve entrapment behind the medial epicondyle. Although this is possible anatomically, patients experiencing pain described as behind the epicondyle are rarely encountered in our experience — no more than three or four in 30 years of acupuncture practice. No acupoint is found behind the epicondyle but one or more are very frequently palpable immediately over it. A cutaneous nerve, the medial antebrachial cutaneous, pierces the deep fascia right at the epicondyle, predisposing the area to sensitivity falsely attributed to the ulnar nerve.

## 12.3.8 Pain in the Forearm (Antebrachium)

The forearm is defined as the region below the elbow and above the proximal crease of the wrist. Pain in the forearm is not common; the most likely place for it to occur is the area adjacent to the lateral border of the cubital fossa, where the median nerve runs under the muscle layer. Injury to muscles of the forearm, such as flexor carpi radialis and pronator teres, is not likely, but if it occurs, branches of the median nerve to the muscles can be damaged and produce pain. Treatment of this pain is relatively straightforward, consisting of placing needles in any tender points. It should not take more than a couple of treatments to treat the pain.

## 12.3.9 Pain in the Wrist

The term *wrist joint* is imprecise anatomically because the wrist area contains 15 bony elements: the distal ends of radius and ulna, eight carpal bones arranged in two rows, and the proximal ends of the five metacarpals. The proximal row of carpal bones consists of the scaphoid (also known as navicular), lunate (or semilunar), and two triquetral bones, one of which is also known as the pisiform. The distal row consists of the trapezium, trapezoid, capitate, and hamate bones. These bones are interconnected by numerous ligaments to form many articulations. The term *wrist joint* often includes all of the articulations among the bones just described. Three nerves — superficial radial, median, and ulnar — pass through the wrist to innervate the hand and fingers. Injuries to the wrist to include all of the joints in the area will manifest as pain along these three nerves.

Pain on the radial side of the wrist may result from injury to the superficial radial nerve from bony or ligamentous injury, or tenosynovitis (e.g., de Quervain's tenosynovitis). The condition of basal arthritis of the thumb is a frequent cause of pain described next in discussion of conditions of the hand. The superficial radial nerve becomes subcutaneous, covered only by skin, at the distal third of the forearm and then runs distally into the web between the thumb and index finger where it forms the Superficial Radial (12) acupoint. In the wrist area, where the superficial radial nerve is only covered by skin, injury can occur relatively easily, resulting in a pain syndrome known clinically as superficial radial neuropathy. Patients often describe such a pain as running along the last 5 to 7 cm of the distal radius into the thumb or its web space.

An example is Lupe, a 53-year-old housewife who caught her hand in a door, resulting in pain in the styloid process along the superficial radial nerve distally to the trapezium. Her pain sensitivity was zero. She did, of course, have a few tender points along the wrist over the styloid process of the radius. Her pain resolved after three treatments that used needles in the primary points and four more along the length of the superficial radial nerve, starting about 7 cm proximal to the styloid process and continuing every 1 to 2 cm to the process. The first treatment was administered to her while she was in the supine position, as was the second; she was in the sitting position for the third treatment.

Similar pain can also result from overuse, as in excessive use of a computer mouse or keyboard. These injuries are often associated with ergonomic issues such as a work surface that is too high for the user. Pain may be perceived along the superficial radial nerve, as above, or across the dorsum of the wrist, in which case needles are placed in a row from the radial styloid to the ulnar styloid, as shown in Figure 12.5. Pain from the superficial radial nerve is subcutaneous, being perceived as being right under the skin. In this setting, needles can be inserted very superficially, approximately half a centimeter deep. On the other hand, pain caused by torn ligaments, bony fractures, and arthritic diseases in the wrist area can be deep and needles will need to penetrate the joint capsule where passive acupoints can be palpated.

Pain on the ulnar side of the wrist occurs infrequently as a result of injury or arthritis at the articulation of the ulna and pisiform or as a result of ulnar neuropathy, possibly resulting from a direct blow, in the same area (where the ulnar nerve becomes superficial). Like superficial radial neuropathy, pain over the ulnar side of wrist is easily managed by placing three or four needles in the area where the pain appears, typically along the lateral border of the hypothenar eminence. Again, how deeply needles are inserted depends on whether the pain is superficial or deep in the joints. This topic is examined further in the discussion of pain in the hand in the next section.

The median nerve in the carpal tunnel under the flexor retinaculum on the palmar surface of the distal forearm is often susceptible to a neuropathy (carpal tunnel syndrome) thought to be caused by compression of the nerve and is often treated with surgical decompression. The condition begins with wrist pain or numbness perceived at the end of a night's sleep; it then progresses to an earlier hour at night and finally affects the sufferer during the day. It may progress to both wrists after a period of time and may result in thenar atrophy and fixed sensory loss in extreme cases. Flexing and extending the wrist aggravates the pain; using wrist splints at night can often reverse the course of the disease if begun early enough. Often the compression results from a flexor tenosynovitis, so a medical treatment for the condition is steroid injection to reduce the inflammation and swelling.

Females are far more often affected than males; their symptoms are often bilateral, while males' are usually unilateral, primarily as result of a direct injury. Ergonomic factors, such as a workstation too high for the user, are thought to contribute to the syndrome; this may explain the predominance of female patients because males are generally taller than females and can tolerate a higher work surface. Factors such as pregnancy, kidney dialysis, diabetes, hypothyroidism, and acromegaly have also been implicated.[9] The authors suspect that low blood pressure and dysmenorrhea are contributing causes in females. Females often develop the condition spontaneously as their pain sensitivity rises to about the four-degree level. The condition is not then hard to manage with acupuncture, but as the pain sensitivity progresses, treatment becomes progressively more difficult. At six degrees, pain is still manageable with needles; at nine, it is very difficult and pain may persist even after surgery is performed to relieve the compression of the nerve. Treatment consists of needling the primary points, plus the Median (U) and the Recurrent of Median (46), while the patient is, first, in the supine, then the prone, and finally the sitting position. The sequence is repeated after a lapse of about a week until symptoms resolve or treatment is abandoned because of lack of response. See Figure 12.6.

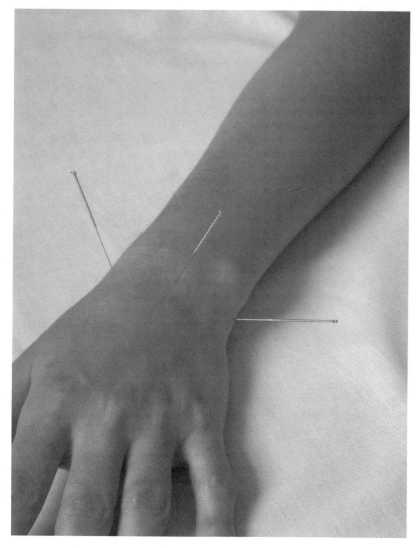

**FIGURE 12.5** Needle locations for treating pain across the dorsum of the wrist. More needles can be added as needed between those shown above.

### 12.3.10 PAIN IN THE HAND

The pain of carpal tunnel syndrome can extend to the hand, as can the pain of the other neuropathies. Sometimes the exact etiology of the pain is uncertain, as in the case of Angela, age 47. She presented complaining of pain around the metacarpophalangeal joint of the left thumb. This could have been arthritic in nature or the result of capsulitis or a superficial radial neuropathy. Her pain sensitivity was four degrees and there were a few passive points around the joint; the dorsal side was tenderer than the ventral. She attributed her pain to a massage she gave to a colleague, during which she used the thumb too much and too hard. A couple of days later, it began to hurt.

Her first acupuncture treatment was administered while she was in the supine position using all accessible primary acupoints, plus four around the joint where tender points were detected. She returned 2 days later for the second treatment and said that the pain in her thumb was reduced substantially. With Angela in the prone position, needles were placed in all accessible primary points plus the same nonspecific acupoints around the joint that were needled previously. She was told to return if the pain recurred.

She returned 3 months later with renewed pain not associated with giving a massage. She then said that she had experienced a similar problem 24 years ago when she picked up a heavy bucket of water too fast and felt pain in her left wrist. At that time she received three injections in her wrist from her doctor and then stopped going back because of the pain of the injections. She then tried an Oriental acupuncturist who gave her nine treatments of two or three needles in the wrist each time, without much relief, although the pain eventually subsided on its own. On this third visit to our clinic the pain had moved to the ventral side of the metacarpophalangeal joint. She received four treatments given over an 8-day period and

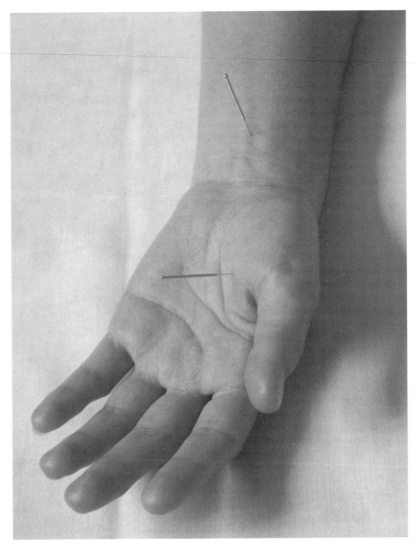

**FIGURE 12.6** Needle locations for treating median neuropathy at the wrist (carpal tunnel syndrome). Additional points along the median nerve can be added as needed.

then was advised to wait a week and return for a reevaluation. When she returned, she was almost pain free.

Pain in the first carpometacarpal joint (sometimes more conveniently called the *basal joint*) is frequently seen and often the source of pain with an uncertain etiology. Arthritis in the joint is common and may progress to the point that fusion or joint replacement may be required. A radial neuropathy or tendinitis may also cause pain around the joint. Inflammation of the three muscles in the thenar compartment (flexor pollicis brevis, abductor pollicis brevis, and opponens pollicis) may also cause pain in the joint. These three muscles have origins in the trapezium or the head of the first metacarpal bone, or both. Often, pain attributed to arthritis responds readily to acupuncture, suggesting that another cause is more likely. When acupuncture is used to address pain in this joint, needles are placed in systemic primary points and tender points around the joint. Needles can also be

applied along the radial nerve as described earlier in discussion of the wrist.

Pain in the palm of the hand may result from carpal tunnel syndrome or Dupuytren's contractures, a fibrosing disorder of unknown origin resulting in development of fibrotic cords or plaques in the palmar aponeurosis along the tendons of flexors digitorum profundus to the third and fourth digits. The treatment is primarily surgical, although topical verapamil is being investigated as a possible alternative. Often the pain does not resolve with surgery, and acupuncture can be used to treat pain before or after a surgical procedure. The acupuncture treatment consists of needling primary points along with affected points in the hand, almost always including those around the third and fourth metacarpophalangeal joints.

Pain in the hypothenar compartment typically follows the course of the ulnar nerve from the wrist. The nerve is bifurcated into two branches — superficial and deep

— with the deep branch going to the muscles in the hypothenar compartment and the superficial branch going to skin over dorsal and ventral surfaces of the ulnar side of the hand. Pain deep inside the hypothenar compartment most likely originates from the deep ulnar nerve or the muscles that it innervates. The pain is treated with three or four needles placed deep enough to reach the muscle layers, and the result usually is good. This type of pain is rarely seen. If the superficial ulnar nerve is involved, cutaneous tingling or numbing pain can be perceived distally, to the little and ring fingers. Such nociceptive sensation will not generate passive acupoints in the fingers, so only points located over the ulnar border of the hand need to be needled.

Pain in the fingers most often results from rheumatoid arthritis or osteoarthritis, the former affecting the proximal interphalangeal joints and the latter the distal joints. (Pain in the interphalangeal joint of the thumb is unusual.) Rheumatoid arthritis can eventually affect the distal interphalangeal joints as well. Deformity and pain are not always well correlated because each can exist without the other; some patients have severe pain with little deformity. The acupuncture treatment of these conditions is to place needles on both sides of the joints. These areas are the first to become passive in the progression of the arthritis because the proper digital nerves run on the sides of the fingers. Smaller terminal branches from the proper digitals course dorsally and ventrally to the cutaneous layer over the joint and, as the condition progresses, passive points appear on the dorsal and ventral sides of the fingers. By then, pain in the fingers is more difficult to manage.

## 12.3.11 Pain Referred from the Visceral Organs

Referred pain is pain perceived at a location remote from its actual cause. Examples are cardiac pain perceived in the left jaw, shoulder, or arm; gall bladder pain perceived in the right shoulder; and pleuritic pain, e.g., pain from diaphragmatic pleurisy, which can be perceived above the clavicle because the diaphragm receives its innervation from the anterior primary rami of C3 through C5, while the clavicular area is innervated by the supraclavicular nerves arising from C3 and C4. Similarly, innervations to the heart come from thoracic splanchnic branches of the first and second intercostal nerves; the first intercostal nerve participates as the lowest segment in forming the brachial plexus that runs medially along the arm and forearm to reach the ulnar side of the hand. This anatomic relationship explains why cardiac pain can be referred to the wrist. The issue of referred pain is considered more fully in the next chapter.

## REFERENCES

1. Dung, H.C. Acupuncture points of the cervical plexus. *Am. J. Chin. Med.* 12:94, 1984.
2. Travell, J.G. and Simons, D.G. *Myofascial Pain and Dysfunction: Trigger Point Manual.* Williams and Wilkins, Baltimore, 1983.
3. Calabro, J.J. Fibromyalgia: chronic aches, diffuse pain. *Med. Student,* March–April 1982; 17–20.
4. Campbell, S.M. Referred shoulder pain. *Postgrad. Med.* 73:193, 1983.
5. Sheon, R.P. et al. *Soft Tissue Rheumatic Pain: Recognition, Management, Prevention.* Lea & Febiger, Philadelphia, 1982.
6. Cailliet, R. *Shoulder Pain,* 5th printing. F.A. Davis Company, Philadelphia, 1973.
7. Burkhead, W.Z. *Rotator Cuff Disorders.* Williams & Wilkins Company, Baltimore, 1996.
8. Rockwood, C.A. and Matsen, F.A. *The Shoulder,* vols. 1 and 2. W.B. Saunders Company, Philadelphia, 1990.
9. Dawson, D.M. et al. *Entrapment Neuropathies.* Little Brown, Boston, 1984.

# 13 Conditions of the Thorax, Abdomen, and Pelvis

## CONTENTS

## 13.1 OVERVIEW

Three issues are more or less unique to the thorax, abdomen, and pelvis. One is pain occurring along a dermatomal distribution, such as that of the post-herpetic syndrome previously discussed in Chapter 11; this dermatomal separation exists because of the lack of interconnections between most spinal nerves of the thoracic spine. Another is the issue of back pain, a major source of disability in the developed world. Finally, interconnections between visceral organs and surface anatomy raise issues of referred pain (briefly mentioned in the previous chapter) and the use of acupuncture to treat visceral problems, most notably asthma. After a discussion of the relevant neuroanatomy, these issues will be explored further.

## 13.2 ACUPUNCTURE AND NEUROANATOMY

Innervation of the thorax, abdomen, and pelvis is supplied by the thoracic, lumbar, sacral, and coccygeal segments of the spine. There are twelve pairs of thoracic spinal nerves, five pairs of lumbar spinal nerves, five pairs of sacral spinal nerves, and three pairs of coccygeal spinal nerves. With the exception of the first thoracic spinal nerves, which participate in the brachial plexus, the thoracic spinal nerves appear to have no interconnections and innervate strict dermatomal patterns. The organization of a typical spinal nerve is shown in Figure 13.1, which illustrates the combination of the dorsal and ventral roots of the spinal cord and subsequent division into two primary rami: anterior (ventral) and posterior (dorsal). Most

ventral primary rami will have two cutaneous nerves from which acupoints can be formed.[1] The cutaneous nerves of ventral primary rami in the thorax and abdomen are known as anterior and lateral cutaneous branches. Dorsal primary rami have muscular and cutaneous branches; the former are generally unnamed.

Each ventral primary ramus has three types of nerve fibers: afferent (sensory); efferent to skeletal muscle; and efferent to cardiac and smooth muscle. Afferent fibers from the ventral primary rami join postganglionic sympathetic fibers at sympathetic trunk ganglia alongside the spinal cord to form splanchnic nerves that innervate the visceral organs, controlling their function (*splanchnic* means visceral, or of the internal organs). In the thorax and abdomen, each ventral primary ramus gives a splanchnic branch. The first four splanchnic branches come from the first four typical spinal nerves (T1 through T4, disregarding fibers that participate in the brachial plexus) and are distributed to organs in the thorax, heart, and lungs. Splanchnics from T5 through T10 join together as the greater splanchnic branch and those from T11 through L3 form the lesser splanchnic. The fourth and fifth lumbar and the first sacral spinal nerves form the least splanchnic. (Nomenclature varies somewhat among authorities.)

The splanchnic nerves serve as an internal connection between acupoints outside and visceral organs inside the body so that it is possible to alter the function of internal organs by stimulating the surface of the body. This is the basis of the so-called cutaneovisceral or viscerocutaneous reflex. If a cold beaker of ice is applied to the abdominal regions, for example, the mucosa of the duodenum constricts and the capillary beds in the villi of the intestine

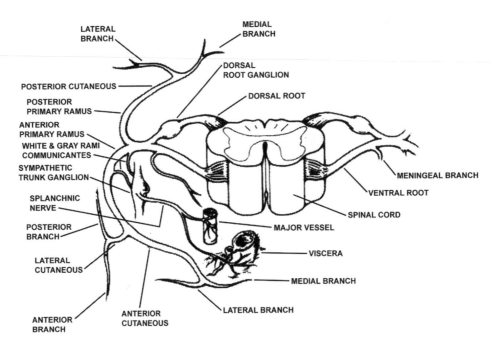

**FIGURE 13.1** Organization of a typical spinal nerve.

become ischemic.[2] This stimulus is transmitted through the spinal nerve to the spinal cord and on to the visceral organs via the splanchnic nerves. Needle stimulation, on the other hand, has been reported not to produce constriction of the arterioles and ischemia in the villi but to produce the opposite effect: vascular dilation in the gastrointestinal tract.[3]

Each ventral primary ramus of the thoracic spinal nerves has muscular and cutaneous branches; the former are rarely used in acupuncture because the intercostal muscles are thin and small and the nerve branches to these muscles are small and deep in the chest wall. Only the cutaneous branches have some practical use. Each ventral primary ramus of a thoracic spinal nerve bifurcates into two branches: the anterior cutaneous and the lateral cutaneous (see Figure 13.2). The anterior cutaneous has two terminal branches but for our purposes can be considered as forming one acupoint to each side of the sternum or the linea alba, depending on the spinal level (see Figure 13.3). The lateral cutaneous nerves also have two terminal branches forming a single acupoint located in the midaxillary line at each spinal level.

In practice, these points are rarely used in acupuncture; they are important because pain or tenderness in these points may originate from visceral organs. This pain may be called referred pain and has also been referred to as the cutaneovisceral reflex or as the viscerocutaneous reflex[2-4] described earlier. One example is the Anterior Cutaneous of T5, located just to the side of the xiphoid process of the sternum, which may become tender in response to chronic stomach problems such as those resulting from the long-term consumption of nonsteroidal anti-inflammatory drugs.

The lumbar plexus is considered generally in the next chapter, but cutaneous nerves and acupoints derived from it, such as the Lateral Cutaneous of L1 (U), Lateral Femoral Cutaneous (U) from L2 and L3, Iliohypogastric (U) from L1, Ilioinguinal (66) from L1, and Genitofemoral (U) from L1 and L2, supply the pelvic area and are therefore described here (see Figure 13.4). The anterior cutaneous of L1 — the iliohypogastric nerve with its associated acupoint, Iliohypogastric (U) — is another example of the viscerocutaneous reflex because it becomes tender during painful menstruation with the contraction of the uterine myometrium that is innervated by splanchnic branches of L1 and L2. This point can also become tender with prostatitis or prostatic enlargement in males. Referred visceral pain may well require a medical investigation into its cause prior to, or along with, providing symptomatic acupuncture intervention.

The Ilioinguinal point is interesting in that it becomes tender in long-standing back pain in older persons, indicating the progression of pathology from lower to upper lumbar levels. It can also become acutely painful if the nerve is injured during surgery to repair an inguinal hernia. The Genitofemoral point is occasionally useful for patients with pain in the scrotum or labium majus; it is actually a pair of points, each located about a centimeter from the anterior border between the skin of the scrotum or labium majus and the skin of the adjacent thigh. One point is on the thigh and the other next to it on the genital skin. This nerve can also be injured during surgery, causing pain in the scrotum or labium majus. The lateral femoral cutaneous nerve is thought by most authorities to be associated with meralgia paraesthetica, a condition of

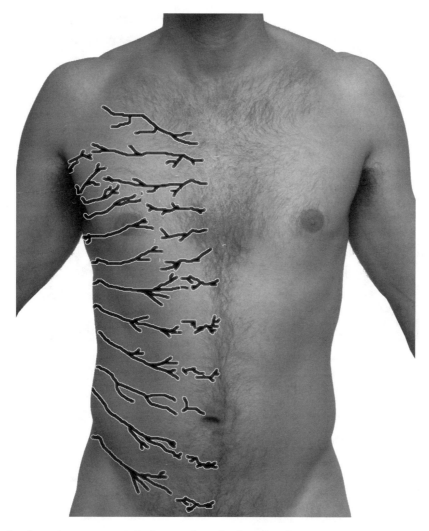

**FIGURE 13.2** Lateral and anterior cutaneous spinal nerves from the thoracic spine.

the lower extremity discussed in the next chapter; its acupoint is rarely tender. Any needling of the points in the inguinal area should be undertaken with care to avoid the femoral artery.

The pudendal nerves arise from the sacral plexus to innervate the genital area and are occasionally treated with acupuncture needles placed 1 to 2 cm deep, just lateral to the labia majora in females or to the scrotum in males. In either case needles are placed approximately in the middle of an anterior–posterior line drawn beside the genitals. The pudendal nerves innervate the anal sphincter, participate in penile erection in males, control the genital muscles, and innervate the vestibular bulb and clitoris in females. Their major use in acupuncture is to control stress urinary incontinence in females. Theoretically, some argument could be made for needling these points in cases of fecal incontinence or impotence, but the authors have little experience in the use of acupuncture for these conditions. Other nerves of the sacral plexus will be considered in more detail in the next chapter.

The lateral cutaneous nerves are sometimes important for another reason — their association with post-herpetic neuralgia, with its pain coursing along the distribution of the thoracic spinal nerves in the intercostal spaces. This area of distribution is known as a *dermatome*, which can be defined as the skin area innervated by a single spinal nerve. Post-herpetic neuralgia in the thorax and abdomen typically involves two to three dermatomes.

Each of the 33 spinal nerves has one dorsal primary ramus generally containing an unnamed muscular branch and a cutaneous branch named as the posterior cutaneous branch of its associated spinal nerve (e.g., "posterior cutaneous of T12"). Generally, each ramus divides into medial and lateral branches, which innervate intrinsic muscles of the neck and back before becoming cutaneous to supply skin. The two branches should properly be called the medial branch of the posterior cutaneous and the lateral branch of the posterior cutaneous, but because the distinction is not important for our purposes, they are grouped together as posterior cutaneous nerves. In the thoracic

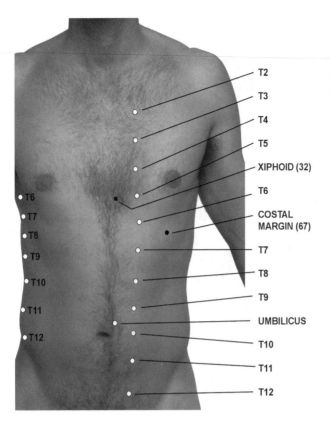

**FIGURE 13.3** Acupoints from the anterior cutaneous spinal nerves, depicted on the model's left side, and some from the lateral cutaneous spinal nerves, shown on the model's right.

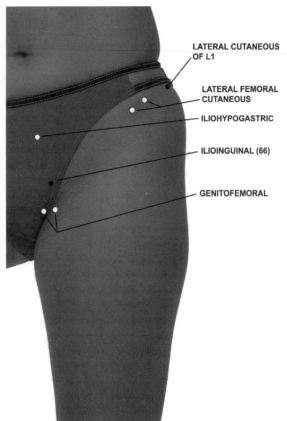

**FIGURE 13.4** Acupoints of the inguinal region formed by cutaneous nerves of the lumbar plexus.

area, the medial branches are larger than the lateral ones; the lateral ones get progressively larger and the medial ones get smaller further down the spine. At the C1 level, there is no cutaneous branch at all and the muscular branch supplies the muscles of the suboccipital triangle, such as the obliquus capitis inferior. Thus, there is no acupoint at this level.

The dorsal primary ramus of C2 is the largest in the body and has already been discussed in Chapter 12 as the greater occipital nerve with its associated acupoint, the Greater Occipital (7). The dorsal primary ramus of C3 was also discussed in the previous chapter as the third occipital nerve and its associated acupoint, the Third Occipital (U). The C4 dorsal primary ramus is very small and probably contributes a few fibers to the brachial plexus; it does not have an associated acupoint. The spinal nerves from C5 through T1 participate in formation of the brachial plexus rather than forming dorsal primary rami and do not have identifiable posterior cutaneous nerves; this explains the dearth of acupoints around the C7 and T1 spinous processes (other than the T1 process).

From T2 through T12, the posterior cutaneous nerves innervate the skin of the back; T6 is the most important of these with its associated acupoint, the Posterior Cutaneous of T6 (21), followed in importance by the Posterior

Cutaneous of T4 (35) and the Posterior Cutaneous of T8 (47). The posterior cutaneous nerves of T2 through T5 are often needled as the "Paravertebral points," especially in the treatment of respiratory conditions such as allergy and asthma, and in smoking cessation. The authors speculate that needling the Paravertebral points may reduce stress because of their close proximity to the sympathetic chain located alongside the spine; they also produce more histaminic reaction than any other points in the body.

Nerves derived from the dorsal primary rami of the lumbar nerves are more complex in their anatomy and nomenclature than those from the thoracic nerves. Fibers from the lateral branches of the dorsal primary rami of the first three lumbar nerves (L1 through L3) combine to form the superior cluneal nerve, with its important Superior Cluneal (14) acupoint that figures prominently in low back pain. The nerve pierces the thoracolumbar fascia at the highest point of the iliac crest to innervate the skin of the gluteal area. The lateral branch of the posterior cutaneous nerve of L2 forms an acupoint — the Posterior Cutaneous of L2 (15); this contrasts with the thoracic area where acupoints are formed by the medial branches of the posterior cutaneous nerves. The lateral branches of the posterior cutaneous nerves emerge superficially along the lateral border of the back muscles known collectively as the erector spinae. The Posterior Cutaneous of L2 (15), located at the waistline, is a frequently used point.

The Posterior Cutaneous of L3 (45) is 2 cm inferior to the L2 point and is a less important acupoint because it is formed by a smaller nerve. The next two dorsal primary rami, L4 and L5, are said to have no cutaneous nerves,[5] possibly because of the large muscle mass of the lumbar muscles requiring the entire contribution of these rami for their innervation. This is one reason that the Posterior Cutaneous of L5 is important in treating low back pain: it is muscular rather than cutaneous. For reasons of convenience and consistency, it is called the Posterior Cutaneous of L5 (22), but it should more properly be called the muscular branch of the posterior primary ramus of L5, as discussed in Chapter 4.

Acupoints associated with posterior cutaneous branches of the five sacral spinal nerves are not generally used in acupuncture, although the Posterior Cutaneous of S3 (104) is a numbered point. The tailbone or coccygeal area can have pain, often severe, affecting the coccygeal posterior cutaneous nerves that are generally grouped together as coccygeal points around, and distal to, the tip of the coccyx. These points are not shown in the accompanying figures because they are normally obscured by gluteal fat. They can be used in conjunction with the pudendal nerve described earlier to treat, for example, stress urinary incontinence.

## 13.3 ACUPUNCTURE APPLIED TO CONDITIONS OF THE THORAX, ABDOMEN, AND PELVIS

Acupuncture in the thorax, abdomen, and pelvis is used primarily to treat musculoskeletal pain such as that associated with acute strains and sprains, herniated intervertebral discs, foraminal stenosis, and facet joint arthritis. Another useful application is the pain remaining after a herpes zoster infection, called post-herpetic neuralgia; this condition follows a strict dermatomal distribution in the thorax and abdomen. Perhaps the most interesting application of acupuncture in the thorax and abdomen (although not particularly useful clinically) is the interaction between the acupoints on the surface of the body and conditions having a visceral origin.

### 13.3.1 MUSCULOSKELETAL PAIN

Low back pain may be the most common condition seen in an acupuncture clinic and is certainly the most important cause of chronic pain. It affects both genders and all ages, and ranges from a dull localized ache to sharp or burning pain radiating down the legs to the feet. It is a condition that may be aggravated by a number of factors ranging from general physical deconditioning and tobacco

consumption to the availability of compensation. Its physical cause is often uncertain despite an extensive work-up. Frequently, psychological components are hard to separate from physical causes. In the acute setting, it responds to nonsteroidal anti-inflammatory drugs (NSAIDs)[6] and advice to stay active;[7] cognitive therapy[2] and multidisciplinary treatment programs[8] may also be helpful.

There have been no randomized controlled trials of acupuncture in the treatment of low back pain, probably because of the difficulty of controlling for the sensation of needle insertion (this problem was discussed in Chapter 1). It has been our experience that low back pain generally responds to acupuncture when pain sensitivity is low. Patients with higher pain sensitivities may also respond, but in most cases the relief is incomplete and temporary. When structural cause of the pain, such as a herniated intervertebral disk, is unresolved, recurrence of symptoms is more likely.

As a general rule, low back pain in patients quantified to have a pain sensitivity of three or less will generally require no more than four treatments to achieve complete resolution of symptoms and those symptoms will probably not recur. When the patient has pain sensitivity between four and six degrees, four to eight treatments will be required to end the pain and the relief may last for years. When the pain sensitivity is seven to nine degrees, it is likely that 8, and possibly as many as 12, treatments will be required to reduce pain to a tolerable level; most of these patients will experience recurrence of pain in a matter of months. Patients with a sensitivity of 10 or higher will usually attain only transient relief after many treatments.

Treatment consists of inserting needles into primary points and points formed by the posterior primary rami in the lumbar distribution. For the patient with a pain sensitivity of three or less, only the primary points need be needled; but as a patient's sensitivity increases, the number of requisite acupoints to be needled correspondingly increases. This regimen follows that generally described throughout this text. Figure 13.5 shows the points in the lumbar area that are typically needled in a patient with low back pain when the patient is in the prone position; this is generally alternated with treatments when he or she is in the supine position with needles placed in the primary acupoints. With pain radiating down either extremity, the patient may also be placed on his or her side with the affected extremity up so that needles may be placed in passive points along its length. When treating a difficult case, as many as six treatment sessions may make up a treatment series: the first should be prone; the second should also be prone and the Posterior Cutaneous of L3 acupoint should be added; the third should be supine; the fourth, prone; the fifth, supine; and the sixth, prone. The side position can be substituted as needed, and the Paravertebral points should be needled once or twice during the series. Then, after a week's rest, treatment series should preferably be limited to three or four sessions.

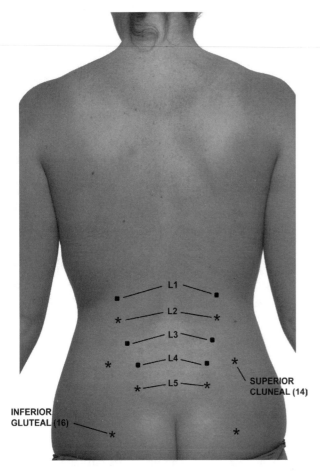

**FIGURE 13.5** The lumbar points typically needled in a patient with low back pain: Superior Cluneal (14); Inferior Gluteal (16); Posterior Cutaneous of L1 (41); Posterior Cutaneous of L2 (15); Posterior Cutaneous of L3 (45); Posterior Cutaneous of L4 (U); Posterior Cutaneous of L5 (22). The Posterior Cutaneous of L1 and Posterior Cutaneous of L3 are used in the more difficult cases.

Two competitive high divers have been seen in the acupuncture clinic and are described here to illustrate the application of acupuncture in back pain. Dan (name has been changed) was completing his bachelor's degree on an athletic scholarship when he began to develop back pain. It was determined that he had mild spondylolisthesis, a forward displacement of one vertebra on another. He had been told by one physician that he would not be able to dive again. He was found to be in the secondary pain category. His back pain was treated with acupuncture in 17 sessions over 2 months while he continued to dive. He was young and healthy, so it should have taken far fewer sessions, but the existence of a structural deficit and his continuing to engage in the activity that produced his pain required more treatment. He became free of pain, however, while he continued to engage in competition diving. Over the following 4 years of college diving, he required 12 more sessions to keep free of pain. Three years after graduating from college, he required one more session to treat

neck pain produced by weight lifting. He was followed up over the next 13 years without any indication of recurrence of pain.

Mike (name has been changed), another diver, sustained an injury of his sacroiliac joint. He was assessed to have a pain sensitivity of four degrees. He began with three treatments utilizing only primary points, the first two were given while he was in the prone position; in the third treatment, he was supine. Then, a short time later, he had four more sessions. It was only after these seven sessions that he was able to resume diving. Over the next 7 years, he required a total of 51 treatments, not just for his back but also for a toe and a wrist. He went on to represent the U.S. in two Olympic games. After ending his diving career, his pain ceased. He became a diving coach and has periodically sent athletes to the clinic for acupuncture treatment of their low back pain.

Once patients are in the tertiary pain category, they require many more treatments and precise needle placement. If they have had prior surgery, they are more difficult to treat and the results are less predictable. It is not unusual for patients to return for treatment hundreds of times. When treating these patients, the acupuncturist should find each individual acupuncture point with fingertip palpation prior to inserting needles. It is important that each patient (regardless of pain sensitivity) feel each of the needles, especially those placed in the Posterior Cutaneous acupoints of L2 (15), L4 (U), and L5 (22), and in the Superior Cluneal (14) acupoints. To needle this last point, it is necessary to direct the point of the needle over the top of the iliac crest and then inferiorly into the nerve; a longer needle than usual may be required in obese patients. Needles up to 6 in. long are available.

An example of a tertiary patient with back pain is Mario, a 57-year-old tile salesman quantified at seven degrees of pain sensitivity. His pain began 40 years earlier when he slipped and fell, and he continued to suffer with it after that incident. He would go to a chiropractor or take acetaminophen, both of which were initially effective. Two and a half weeks before his first visit to the acupuncture clinic, he was reaching up to change a light bulb and felt a sharp exacerbation of the pain. Neither the chiropractor nor the acetaminophen helped. A cousin suggested that he come for acupuncture, but he delayed seeking treatment because he lived 3 hours from the clinic.

When Mario finally came, he had some relief immediately after the first treatment, administered when he was in the prone position. The next two treatments were administered while Mario was in the supine, then the prone, positions, and after these three treatments he experienced sufficient relief that he did not return to the clinic for 11 months. At that time, he related that during that lapse he had fallen while mowing his yard and had been caught by the blade of the lawnmower, fracturing several ribs. Yet, after that episode he had no pain at all for nearly

3 months until he began having right-sided headaches and right neck and shoulder pain. At first the headaches and musculoskeletal pain were effectively managed with acetaminophen and muscle relaxants, but a month later the pills were no longer helping and Mario came back to the acupuncture clinic for treatment.

He related that each day the pain would start in the morning at the area of the right dorsal scapular nerve and then extend as the day progressed to the greater occipital area. He was placed on his left side and needles were placed in the primary and secondary points from the dorsal scapular to the greater occipital down to the arms, forearms, and hands. In the other areas, only primary acupoints were treated. Because of the distance he had to travel, Mario was needled each of the following 2 days; the second treatment in this series was administered while he was in the prone position and for the third he was in the supine position, with the same strategy followed in each session.

Mario presented to the clinic 2 months later as an emergency after reinjuring his back attempting to lift a heavy gas tank. He was given 14 needles in the lumbar area, including three pairs of secondary acupoints; this proved to be too many, causing a flare-up of pain. He came to the clinic the next day with a crutch because he was having difficulty walking. He was treated in the prone position again with only eight needles placed in the lumbar area. He did not appear at the clinic until 4 years later, when his back flared up again and he came for another series of three treatments. He said at that time that his back had not bothered him during those 4 years.

Female patients whose pain sensitivities are 10 or more are very likely to develop intractable back pain. These women almost certainly have had years of dysmenorrhea. Their pain may be diminished with acupuncture, but only temporarily. Men too can have high sensitivities, although the causes are more varied. Sadly, some of these patients have had several hundred visits to the acupuncture clinic for temporary and incomplete pain relief.

It is rare for the pain sensitivity level in patients to fall over time, although some amount of day-to-day fluctuation is possible. Systemic illness may elevate pain levels. When a profound reduction in pain sensitivity does occur, it raises questions about the validity of the earlier, higher assessment. A confounding factor in assessing pain, previously mentioned, is prior back surgery. Jay, a 50-year-old dentist, is one patient whose pain sensitivity dropped over several years. When he was initially seen for back pain after he had undergone four surgeries, he was measured to have a sensitivity of seven. He had some relief of his back pain after 28 acupuncture treatments. He returned for three more treatments 2 years later and was reassessed to have a sensitivity of only five.

Joan, a 40-year-old psychotherapist, illustrates another cause of back pain. She began having pain in her coccyx subsequent to back surgery for degenerative disks;

this presentation of coccygeal pain occurring after back surgery is not uncommon. She also complained of pain in her hips and pelvis and related that she had a sleep disorder and was taking hydrocodone, prednisone, and sulindac because she had been diagnosed with an autoimmune connective tissue disorder. She was assessed to have a pain sensitivity of seven degrees. Her back, hip, and pelvis pain resolved after 12 treatments administered over approximately 2 months.

Another cause of back pain is a direct blow to the coccyx. These injuries can be very painful and can include coccygeal fracture. Obviously, the outcome is better in the absence of fracture. Needles are placed in the skin innervated by the posterior primary rami of the five sacral nerves and the first coccygeal spinal nerve under the tip of the tailbone (the needle is angled upward), as well as points formed by the inferior gluteal, pudendal, obturator, ilioinguinal, genitofemoral, and iliohypogastric nerves, depending on the patient's position. For example, in the prone position, acupoints representing the posterior primary rami of sacral and coccygeal spinal nerves, inferior gluteal nerves, and pudendal nerves are needled. In the supine position, acupoints of the pudendal, obturator, ilioinguinal, genitofemoral, and iliohypogastric nerves are needled. In the setting of fracture, exceptional care should be taken to avoid introducing bacteria into the fracture site (although we have never had a problem with infection).

Postoperative pain in the chest deserves special mention because it is frequently encountered. Pain after open-heart surgery persists long after the skin has healed and is easily treated with acupuncture. Breast implants also may present with ongoing pain. Abdominal surgery patients may present with pain and tenderness around their surgical wounds. In each case, treatment consists of placing needles around the margin of the painful area; it is futile to place needles directly into scars, which are insensitive. Obviously, with breast implants, it is imperative to avoid placing needles into the implants, and at least one of the authors regularly queries all his new female patients as to the presence of implants before placing needles in the lateral pectoral or medial pectoral acupoints or into any other acupoints that may lie over an implant. With the increasing prevalence of other types of implants such as pacemakers, pumps, and shunts, the practitioner should always be aware of their existence and location before planning acupuncture treatment; in many cases these devices are obvious on inspection, but by far the safest route is to query patients beforehand about their presence.

### 13.3.2 DERMATOMAL PAIN

Of course, the lower back is not the only source of pain. The mid- and upper back, ribs, intercostal muscles, costochondral junctions, and abdominal wall muscles are subject to contusions, fractures, strains, and sprains. The principles of treatment should sound familiar: place needles nonspecifically around the site of pain and along its dermatomal innervation, targeting the posterior, lateral, and anterior cutaneous nerves in particular; add needles to primary, secondary, and tertiary points as necessary, depending on the patient's pain sensitivity, response to treatment, and tolerance of needling.

If begun early, acupuncture is effective in the treatment of pain that frequently accompanies herpes zoster (shingles) and then remains after the infection and rash have subsided. As previously mentioned, shingles is the manifestation of reactivation of the varicella virus, which causes chicken pox.[9] After an episode of chicken pox has remitted, the virus migrates and hides in the trigeminal[10] and dorsal root ganglia.[11] It remains dormant in the ganglia until immunological weakness in the host provides an opportunity for the virus to reactivate and migrate down the axons to cause the characteristic rash and pain — sometimes followed by post-herpetic neuralgia after the rash has resolved. One cause of the causative immunological weakness is simply age and, accordingly, herpes often affects seniors. In our clinic, we have also seen some younger patients with high pain sensitivities with this condition. We have had older patients of low degree, e.g., two or three, who have had shingles without any ensuing neuralgia. This leads us to speculate that the neuralgia is more likely to appear in higher-degree patients.

We have also found that the neuralgia is easier to treat with acupuncture if it has not been long-standing. We suspect that once the virus traverses the length of the axon, it causes a retrograde destruction of the nerve's myelin sheath back to the sensory neurons in the ganglia. We further speculate that one effect of acupuncture may be to promote remyelination. If our speculations are correct, it would follow that once retrograde destruction is complete, for example, after a year or so, the myelin sheath has little chance of regenerating and thus the chance that acupuncture can help is small.

To apply the general principles of treatment to the post-herpetic neuralgia patient, needles would be placed in primary and probably some secondary and tertiary points, along with a line of needles spaced every 2 to 3 cm around the periphery of the rash; if islands of unaffected skin are within the general area of the rash, needles could be placed there also. These needles should be placed superficially, especially in thin patients, to avoid causing a pneumothorax. It is beneficial to place needles in the posterior, lateral, and anterior cutaneous points corresponding to the dermatomal distribution of the pain, to the extent possible without actually placing needles into the rash. The side position is particularly appropriate in these cases because the distribution of the nerve can be followed from the spine to the patient's anterior surface. In summary, as mentioned earlier, it is important to begin soon enough — within a year of the onset of symptoms

— and success is largely predicted by the degree of pain sensitivity of the patient.

One condition that mimics post-herpetic neuralgia in a small handful of patients is that of pleurodynia — pain caused by an excessive accumulation of fluids in the costodiaphragmatic recess, especially during the day when the recess is dependent. The fluids press on the intercostal nerves in the T7 and T8 distribution, causing pain. The pain of pleurodynia is perceived in the costal arch as dull and achy while post-herpetic neuralgia pain is described as sharp and burning and can occur in a variety of dermatomes. Pleurodynia pain is normally reduced at night when the patient is lying flat. The source of the fluid requires a medical investigation. The pain is easily managed in one to three sessions, emphasizing the placement of 12 to 16 needles along the costal arch in the first treatment with the patient supine, and along the T7 and T8 intercostal space in the second treatment with the patient in the prone position; if a third treatment is required the more painful side should be positioned up and needles placed along the intercostal space from the spine to the associated anterior cutaneous acupoints. Of course, in each session, primary and secondary points, particularly in the upper half of the body, are also needled. The needles in the chest wall should be placed as deep as possible without piercing the pleural cavity.

The term *costochondritis* implies pain at the costochondral junction, that is, the connection formed between the cartilaginous and bony portions of ribs near their sternal junction; however, in our experience this pain and tenderness most often occur at the junction of the cartilage and the sternum. They are fairly easily treated with needles in the affected areas. Because of some concern that this pain may actually reflect a viscerocutaneous reflex from the heart, a cardiac evaluation should be considered.

### 13.3.3 Viscerocutaneous Interaction

The relationship between the skin surface and the organs within is a truly fascinating subject, one that could easily lead to extravagant claims about acupuncture. The role of the splanchnic nerves and their interaction with the cutaneous nerves at the spinal cord was introduced previously. It may be possible to change the functioning of internal organs through needle stimulation of points on the skin in the same dermatome, but in most cases better treatments are available for pathological conditions of these organs. Also, the duration of acupuncture's effects in these settings is highly variable. Acupuncture *can* ameliorate gastric discomfort and pain resulting from hyperacidity, for example, but certainly more convenient and predictable pharmacological solutions exist.

Conversely, the existence of this interconnection may have diagnostic significance, but in the developed world no responsible physician would make a diagnosis on this evidence alone. Tenderness of acupoints around the xiphoid process of the sternum may help distinguish a noncardiac source of chest pain (e.g., dyspepsia) from one of myocardial origin, but surely an electrocardiogram is more reliable. (Temporal issues come into play in this setting because the xiphoid points could be tender in the face of long-standing gastric pain, but points in the chest wall would probably not become tender instantaneously in the setting of an acute cardiac event.)

However, there is little doubt that the connection exists and, if for nothing more than intellectual curiosity, it is noteworthy. Occasionally, as in the case of bronchial asthma and allergy, it is useful in cases that are refractory to pharmacological intervention. Patients suffering these conditions, among them a 7-year-old boy named Randall, are noteworthy in that they have a great number of passive acupoints in the thorax, particularly along the clavicles, sides of the trachea, and the sternal border (the latter representing the anterior cutaneous nerves). Randall was the youngest patient ever seen in the acupuncture clinic. His mother wanted him to try acupuncture to see if it was possible to control the asthmatic attacks that he had suffered so frequently since his infancy. Not too long before he came in, he had almost drowned in a river not far from the family ranch. Although it was midsummer, the water in the river was still very cold, so cold that when Randall jumped in, he was not able to breathe because, as he described it, his chest became so tight that he was immediately choked up and almost suffocated. He looked weak and seemed underweight for his age.

It was surprising how many passive acupoints were discovered in this boy. All of the points categorized in the primary and secondary groups were in the passive phase, and even some of the tertiary and nonspecific groups were passive, particularly the points in the neck and thorax, the latter representing the anterior, lateral, and posterior cutaneous branches of the upper four thoracic spinal nerves. No such passive points were found outside the neck and thorax. Treatment for asthma is fairly simple: the first three sessions are exactly the same as described in Chapter 11 for sinus allergy. If the patient fails to respond, a careful search should be undertaken for passive acupoints along the clavicles and sides of the trachea; these points can be needled as long as great care is taken not to pierce the vascular structures in the anterior triangle of the neck.

Sam, 73, is another patient who represents an infrequently encountered problem: chronic cough. Although usually trivial, cough can become chronic and incessant; this usually happens because the nerve responsible for the cough reflex — the internal branch of the superior laryngeal located under the mucosa of the piriform recess — is damaged because of disease or trauma. Irritation to the mucosa will generate a cough reflex. Despite an extensive work-up, no cause had been found for Sam's cough, which

had begun more than 2 years earlier after coronary bypass surgery. He had no pain anywhere, but his sensitivity was a rather high eight degrees. His treating acupuncturist speculated that the surgery damaged his vagus nerve and that this in turn damaged the superior laryngeal. The suspicion was based on the fact that his anterior cervical area was very sensitive upon palpation, particularly in the area inferior to the hyoid bone where the internal branch of the superior laryngeal nerve runs through the infrahyoid muscle. He would cough when the area was pressed with a finger.

Sam came for a total of 14 treatments. By his 12th visit, his coughing had substantially decreased. His treatment regimen was very similar to that for patients with headache, or shoulder and neck pain. For the first treatment, he was in the supine position and only primary acupoints were used. For the second treatment (again limited to primary points), he was prone. For the third he was sitting, and the primary and secondary acupoints in the neck, shoulder, and upper limbs were used. During the fourth treatment, he was supine again. This time, in addition to the primary points, four more points, including the cervical plexus and three transverse cervical points, were also used. The fifth treatment took place while he was prone; the primary and Paravertebral points were used. After a 1-week interval, Sam returned for a set of five more treatments, repeating the same five treatments of the first set with the exception that more needles were used in the cervical and supraclavicular regions. The authors have no theoretical basis to explain the effectiveness of acupuncture in this patient.

Conditions in the abdomen may find symptomatic relief from acupuncture. Hiatal hernia is one example. This hernia appears as a localized pain limited to a small area below the xiphoid process at the inferior end of the sternum and is a clear example of viscerocutaneous reflex pain. The esophageal–gastric junction at the diaphragmatic hiatus is innervated by the splanchnic branch of the fifth thoracic spinal nerve, the dermatome of which includes the area of the xiphoid process. Therefore, an irritation in the cardiac portion of the stomach can and does refer pain at the lowest end of the sternum. Better medical treatment of excess gastric secretions and the availability of less irritating over-the-counter analgesics in recent years has reduced the number of acupuncture patients seeking help for this condition, but it remains an interesting anatomical phenomenon.

Similarly, pain from low-grade inflammation or small stones in the gall bladder can be treated with a couple of needles at the lowest point of the costal arch in the T6 dermatome. Patients with bowel disorders such as Crohn's disease, ulcerative colitis, and irritable bowel syndrome (the nomenclature varies somewhat) may benefit from acupuncture as part of a comprehensive approach. Vague gastrointestinal complaints, with uncertain causes despite extensive work-ups, may be relieved by acupuncture, most likely because of increased parasympathetic tone and a resulting normalization of gastrointestinal motility. Pain from adhesions from previous abdominal surgeries may also respond to needles.

Emesis, such as that associated with cancer chemotherapy, has been confirmed by the National Institutes of Health[12] and others[13,14] as an appropriate application for acupuncture. Two points to be included with a basic protocol are the Median (U), approximately 4 cm proximal to the proximal crease of the wrist on the anterior surface of the forearm, and the Common Peroneal-I (24). The Median point is thought to have some cutaneovisceral splanchnic interconnections with thoracic organs and the common peroneal is thought to have such interconnections with the lumbosacral splanchnic branches to the descending and sigmoid colon. These interconnections may explain a mechanism by which acupuncture modifies the activity of digestive organs, or it may be that a generalized increase in parasympathetic tone may account for the role of acupuncture in controlling emesis. Certainly, more research is needed in this important area. The nausea and vomiting of early pregnancy is another condition that may respond well to acupuncture, but the authors are concerned that the hormonal changes produced by needling may cause miscarriages to occur and thus pregnancy is considered by us to be a contraindication to acupuncture.

Pelvic conditions deserve special mention because acupuncture has shown efficacy for a number of them. Before discussing them individually, some general empirical observations are in order. In female patients, acupuncture has unmistakable effects on sex hormones; to some extent, pain sensitivity appears to be a reflection of circulating hormones. As described previously, women are generally more sensitive during menstruation because they complain of needle pain more at that time than at others. The Iliohypogastric point is a sentinel point that is much more likely to be tender during menstruation. The authors have not studied serial pain sensitivities in women and compared them with their menstrual histories, but that would be an easy and interesting study to carry out. Females of reproductive age are often noted to have strong mood disturbances during acupuncture sessions that resolve as soon as the needles are removed; the authors feel this is almost certainly hormonally induced.

Dysmenorrhea is one complaint that demands intervention. It has been seen throughout this text that continuing menstrual pain is a major cause (if not *the* major cause) of increased pain sensitivities later in a woman's life. These high pain sensitivities have major implications for the quality of life as individuals age, in that they reflect or predict refractoriness in pain management. Menstrual cramping must be addressed, not ignored. Young females still at low pain sensitivities but suffering from dysmenorrhea are easily treated pharmacologically (typically with oral contraceptives), with acupuncture, or, in extreme cases, surgically.

The acupuncture treatment is quite effective in low-degree women and consists of nine sessions: each of the sessions involves simple needling of primary points while varying positions as convenient. The third treatment of a set is often done with the patient in the sitting position with needles placed in primary, and also secondary, points. The timing of the sessions is most important: three sessions are performed 2 to 3 days apart in the week before menstruation, and these three sessions are then repeated as needed before the next two menstrual periods. It is not necessary to needle any specific points in the pelvic or inguinal area, although in refractory cases these points could be included without harm. This treatment is almost always effective. For a physician to fail to address a complaint of menstrual cramping in a patient seems to be a disservice to the patient.

Treatment of infertility is another area in which acupuncture shows promise. Author Dung has attempted acupuncture for infertility in 16 females over his career; of these, seven (44%) have had at least one healthy birth after becoming pregnant soon after acupuncture treatments; three did not and six were lost to follow-up. These were difficult cases because the women had tried virtually every other available intervention before turning to acupuncture. The treatment regimen is the same as for dysmenorrhea (described earlier) except that the groups of three sessions are administered in the week prior to ovulation rather than in the week prior to menstruation.

Although this series is too small to justify expansive conclusions, it might be worthwhile for primary care physicians at least to try acupuncture before referring their patients for expensive gynecological procedures. Certainly, this is an area that merits further research. (The authors have no experience with using acupuncture in the treatment of male causes of infertility, but it seems reasonable to attempt a therapeutic trial of both members of the couple before attempting even the most basic work-up. This avoids a determination of "fault" and a work-up that can be embarrassing. The male could be treated at the same time as the female.)

Impotence is another problem for which acupuncture may be useful. (One problem in evaluating the effect of needles on this problem is that a major component of impotence is the presence of psychological issues — a patient's belief that a procedure will help his impotence may be enough in the absence of any physiological effect.) The rationale for using acupuncture in this setting is that, anatomically, one cause of impotence is the inability of the corpora cavernosum to fill with blood to maintain an erection. This mechanism is controlled by the perineal branches of the pudendal nerve. We have found impotent men to have passive acupoints at the location where the pudendal nerve emerges through the pudendal canal medial to the ischial tuberosity. The genitofemoral nerve may also play a role in that it is distributed to the pubic area. Men with impotence also have passive points over the skin superior to symphysis pubis. Additionally, the coccyx has neurological connections with the genital area.

To treat impotence, needles are placed in primary points and at the location of the pudendal nerve to either side of the scrotum and the tip of the coccyx with the patient in the prone position (access is easier if the patient draws his knees up under his chest). They are placed over the superior pubic and inguinal areas, utilizing the Iliohypogastric, Ilioinguinal and Genitofemoral acupoints, when the patient is in the supine position. Response is unpredictable and does not seem to correlate with pain sensitivity, with many patients reporting increased frequency and duration of erections. The effect may initially last a week or two and may be prolonged with repeated treatments. If no effect is seen after about four treatments, acupuncture should be abandoned. Of course, an effective pharmacological treatment for this condition is available, but it is contraindicated in some patients and also expensive. However, if not contraindicated, it may be a better first choice; in difficult cases, both treatments can be administered simultaneously.

Incontinence is yet another area in which acupuncture can be beneficial. The innervation and associated acupoints are the same as for impotence, and the treatment is the same for males and females. Some patients have reported unintended improvement in their incontinence while being treated for other conditions. The duration of improvement is another question the authors are unprepared to answer without further research.

Generally, the iliohypogastric, ilioinguinal, genitofemoral, and obturator nerves may become tender to palpation in the setting of problems or diseases in the urogenital organs, such as prostatitis, vaginal herpes, incontinence, impotence, and others. Because they innervate the areas surrounding the external genitalia, the dermatome of L1 and L2 over the symphysis pubis may also become tender. Needling acupoints in these areas can provide symptomatic relief for these problems and diseases.

In summarizing the fascinating topic of viscerocutaneous interaction, it is important to conclude that patients often present with painful conditions that require medical and surgical interventions. Acupuncture can be beneficial for the accompanying pain once the patient has been started on a plan of definitive treatment that has been well thought out. Other patients have conditions for which the indicated medical and surgical treatments may provide symptomatic relief but have adverse aspects of being poorly tolerated, inconvenient, expensive, contrary to religious or metaphysical beliefs, etc. In these patients, acupuncture may be a wholly satisfactory alternative. Primary care physicians who are prepared to offer this alternative offer a real service to their patients.

## REFERENCES

1. Dung, H.C. Acupuncture points of the typical spinal nerves. *Am. J. Chin. Med.* 13:39, 1985.
2. Kuntz, A. and Haselwood, L.A. Circulatory reactions in the gastro-intestinal tract elicited by local cutaneous stimulation. *Am. Heart J.* 20:743, 1940.
3. Lee, G.T.L. A study of electrical stimulation of acupuncture locus Tsusanli (St.-36) on mesenteric circulation. *Am. J. Chin. Med.* 2:53, 1974.
4. Kuntz, A. Anatomic and physiologic properties of cutaneo-visceral vasomotor reflex. *Arch. J. Neurophysiol.* 8:421, 1945.
5. Woodburne, R.T. *Essentials of Human Anatomy,* 6th ed. Oxford University Press, New York, 1978.
6. Van Tulder, M.W., Koes, B.W., and Bouter, L.M. Conservative treatment of acute and chronic nonspecific low back pain: a systematic review of randomized controlled trials of the most common interventions. *Spine* 22:2128–2156, 1997.
7. Waddell, G., Feder, G., and Lewis, M. Systematic reviews of bed rest and advice to stay active for acute low back pain. *Br. J. Gen. Pract.* 47:647–652, 1997.
8. Karjalainen, K., Malmivaara, A., van Tulder, M., et al. Multidisciplinary biopsychosocial rehabilitation for subacute low back pain among working age adults (Cochrane Methodology Review). In: The Cochrane Library, Issue 4, 2001. Chichester, OK: John Wiley & Sons, Ltd.
9. Dyck, P.J. et al. *Peripheral Neuropathy*, 2nd ed., Vol. I and Vol. II. W.B. Saunders Company, Philadelphia, 1984.
10. Nesburn, A.A. et al. Latent herpes simplex virus. Isolation from rabbit trigeminal ganglia between episodes of recurrent ocular infection. *Arch. Ophthalmol.* 88:412, 1972.
11. Stevens, J.G. and Cook, M.L. Latent herpes simplex virus in spinal ganglia of mice. *Science*, 173:843, 1971.
12. NIH Consensus Conference: acupuncture. *JAMA* 280:1518, 1998 .
13. Dundee, N.W. et al. Acupuncture to prevent cisplatin-associated vomiting. *Lancet* 1:1083, 1987.
14. Shen, J. et al. Electroacupuncture for control of myeloablative chemotherapy-induced emesis. *JAMA* 284:2755, 2000.

# 14 Conditions of the Lower Extremity

## CONTENTS

## 14.1 OVERVIEW

Painful conditions in the lower extremities generally result from direct trauma, wear and tear of weight-bearing joints, and from problems of the lumbar spine causing radiating pain down one or both legs. Lumbar spine issues were discussed in the previous chapter. The feet are another source of lower extremity pain for two reasons: they bear the weight of the entire body over a very small surface, and they are susceptible to circulatory and neurological problems often associated with inactivity, aging, smoking, alcoholism, and diabetes. Bursitis around the greater trochanter and the knee is an inflammatory condition that often can be helped with acupuncture. After a discussion of the relevant anatomy, the acupuncture treatment of these conditions will be examined.

## 14.2 ACUPUNCTURE AND NEUROANATOMY OF THE LOWER EXTREMITY

Innervation of the lower extremities is provided by the lumbar plexus and the sacral plexus. The relationship between these two is similar to that of cervical plexus and brachial plexus in that spinal nerves from the two have a small degree of overlap. Consequently, areas of innervation can become redundant, making clear division of the anatomic topography occasionally difficult. Acupoints

formed by the lumbar plexus[1] and the sacral plexus[2] were first reported in 1985.

### 14.2.1 THE LUMBAR NERVE PLEXUS

Each of the five lumbar spinal nerves divides into two primary rami: the anterior (ventral) and the posterior (dorsal). The anterior primary rami from L1 through L4 interconnect to form the lumbar nerve plexus. Six peripheral nerves arising from the lumbar spinal plexus (shown in Figure 14.1) contribute to the formation of acupoints in the inguinal area, pelvis, anterior and medial compartments of the thigh, and medial surface of the leg. These acupoints in the inguinal and pelvic area are shown in Figure 14.2 and those in the thigh and leg are shown in Figure 14.3a and Figure 14.3b. These points were also discussed in the previous chapter. The anterior primary ramus of L1 splits into three branches: the upper branch becomes the iliohypogastric nerve; the middle branch becomes the ilioinguinal nerve; and the lower branch joins with a branch of the anterior primary ramus of L2 to form the genitofemoral nerve.

The iliohypogastric nerve runs inside the posterior abdominal wall and penetrates the three abdominal muscles to reach the superficial fascia at the pelvic area at a site superior to the spermatic cord and lateral to the suspensory ligament of the penis in the male, and superior to the round ligament and lateral to the suspensory ligament

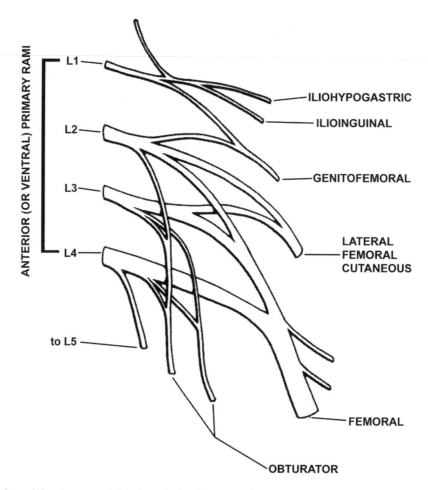

**FIGURE 14.1** The six peripheral nerves arising from the lumbar nerve plexus.

of the clitoris in the female. Where the nerve pierces the deep fascia of the abdomen or anterior layer of the rectus sheath, a rarely used acupoint is formed.

The course of the ilioinguinal nerve is parallel to that of the iliohypogastric. When the ilioinguinal nerve reaches the inguinal region, it passes through the inguinal canal and emerges through the superficial inguinal ring to become the Ilioinguinal (66) acupoint. The point is superficial to the inguinal ring along the inguinal ligament immediately lateral to the tendon of the pectineal muscle at the superior border of the femoral triangle. This is not an important acupoint, except that it is often seen in individuals over the age of 65, thus indicating long-standing lumbar spine disease. Lumbar spine problems tend to begin at the L4 or L5 level and then spread upward and downward; by the time the L1 level is affected, the entire lumbar spine typically shows signs of degeneration.

Branches of the genitofemoral nerve pierce the deep fascia immediately below the inguinal ligament and lateral to the superficial inguinal ring. The genitofemoral nerve divides into two terminal branches: femoral and genital. The genital branch supplies nerve fibers to the scrotum or labia majora and its acupoint is rarely used, primarily because this anatomical area rarely experiences pain (please refer to the previous chapter for a more complete discussion).

The lateral femoral cutaneous nerve is typically described as deriving

> … from the first three lumbar nerves to course across the anterior surface of the iliacus muscle where the muscle forms a part of the wall of the false pelvis and enters the thigh between the lateral border of the iliacus and the upper end of the inguinal ligament. Thereafter it pierces the fascia lata,* commonly just below and medial to the anterior superior iliac spine. The larger part of the nerve runs downward on the lateral side of the anterior aspect of the thigh to supply skin here as far as the knee. A smaller posterior branch runs more laterally, supplying skin below the greater trochanter but usually not reaching the knee.[3]

---

* The fascia lata is the deep fascia wrapping around the muscle mass of the thigh; on the lateral side, it is thickened and known as the iliotibial tract, an extension of the aponeurosis enclosing the tensor fasciae latae muscle.

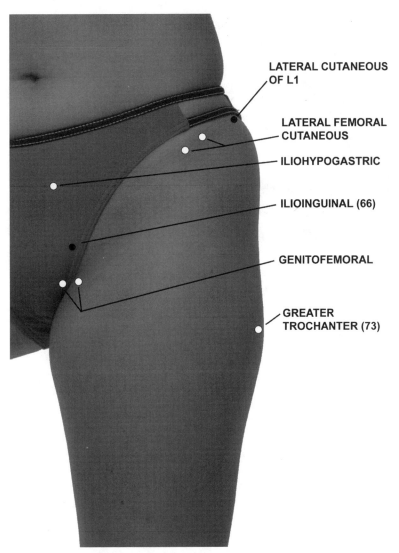

LATERAL CUTANEOUS
OF L1

LATERAL FEMORAL
CUTANEOUS

ILIOHYPOGASTRIC

ILIOINGUINAL (66)

GENITOFEMORAL

GREATER
TROCHANTER (73)

**FIGURE 14.2** Acupoints in the inguinal area arising from the lumbar plexus. The greater trochanter (73) acupoint is also shown, although it is most likely derived from the sciatic nerve plexus.

The nerve is generally thought to be the source of an important problem: meralgia paraesthetica, or "Bernhardt's disease." Some sources have described the lateral femoral cutaneous nerve as the external cutaneous branch of the femoral nerve,[4] but as can be seen from Figure 14.1, it is not a branch of the femoral nerve at all. Careful dissection of the fascia lata, furthermore, reveals that no branches of the nerve penetrate it to become cutaneous although branches penetrate the iliotibial tract directly from the sciatic nerve. The authors' opinion is that the sciatic nerve is more likely responsible for meralgia paraesthetica. This observation remains to be confirmed by other anatomists. If it is true that the lateral femoral cutaneous nerve is not the cause of meralgia paraesthetica, the nerve has little relevance to acupuncture; its acupoint, shown in Figure 14.2, rarely becomes tender, and that fact alone suggests that the nerve is not involved in meralgia paraesthetica.

The largest branch of the lumbar nerve plexus is the femoral nerve. It enters the lower limb by passing under the inguinal ligament deep in the femoral triangle. The femoral nerve sends several cutaneous branches to the skin of the anterior surface of the thigh, as well as muscular branches to the muscles of the anterior compartment of the thigh. A number of acupoints are found in the anterior surface of the thigh (Figure 14.3a and Figure 14.3b). These are formed at sites where the cutaneous branches pierce the deep fascia or at locations of the neuromuscular attachments formed between the muscular branches of the femoral nerve and the muscles of the anterior compartment of the thigh.

These points are relatively unimportant because they do not appear very often. Occasionally, however, it is possible to locate a few detectable acupoints in this area, for example, in individuals suffering a severe crushing injury of the thigh muscles. In this example, internal

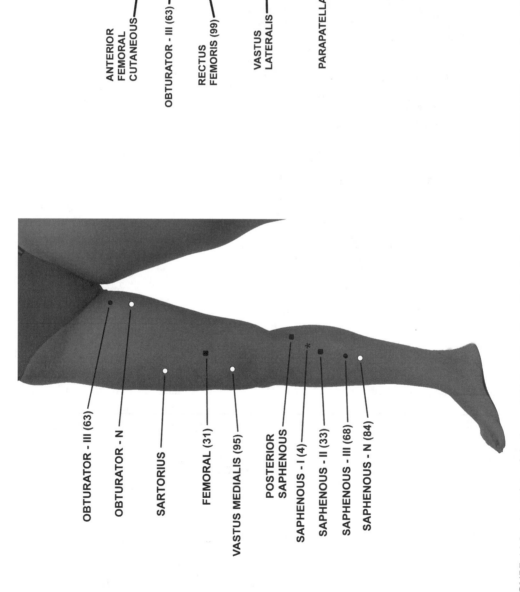

**FIGURE 14.3a** Acupoints of the leg and thigh arising from the lumbar plexus: antero-medial view.

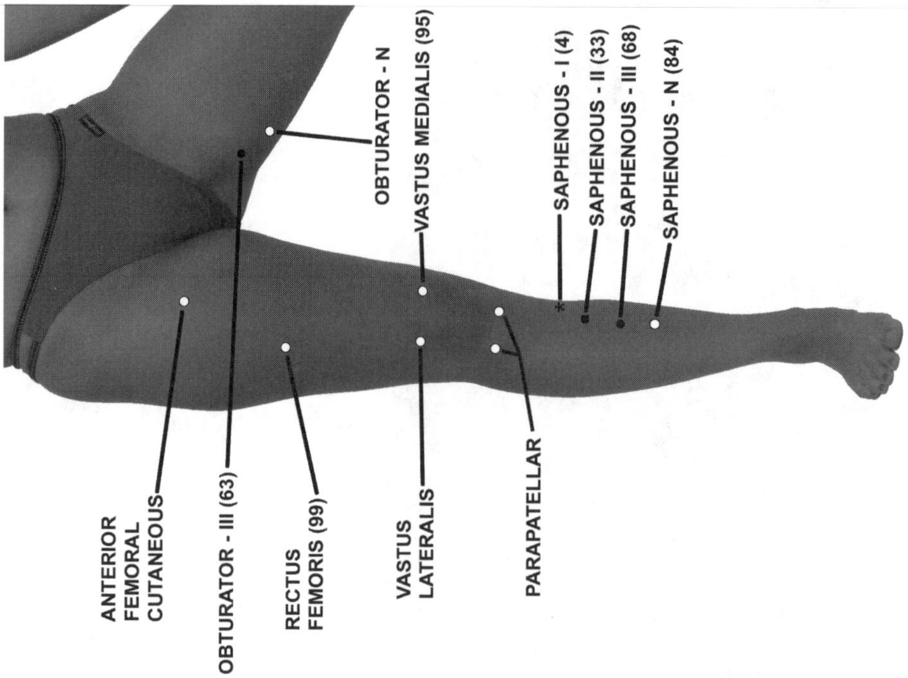

**FIGURE 14.3b** Acupoints of the leg and thigh arising from the lumbar plexus: anterior view.

bleeding due to major vascular damage will occur, and the hematoma formed will take months to subside. Such individuals will be likely to develop chronic pain in the thigh and it becomes possible to palpate their tender acupoints. Another example is elderly individuals who suffer long durations of chronic pain that develops into the allodynic stage, with discomfort and aches in practically all parts of the body; they also are likely to present with tender acupoints on the anterior surface of the thigh. Unfortunately, because of their high pain sensitivities, it is not possible to manage the pain of such patients, so whether one can find any acupoints in the area becomes irrelevant.

Once the femoral nerve courses downward in the medial surface of the thigh and enters the adductor (or Hunter's) canal, it emerges inferomedially from underneath the sartorius muscle, becoming very superficial just immediately below the medial side of the knee under the medial condyle of the tibia. As the nerve pierces the deep fascia at the medial side of the knee, it changes its name to become the saphenous nerve, which is the cutaneous branch. From an acupuncture perspective, the saphenous nerve and its acupoints are the most important components of the lumbar nerve plexus. This cutaneous nerve has branches that innervate the medial surface of the leg as

far as the medial malleolus. Most of its branches are at its proximal end where the nerve penetrates the deep fascia. The area on the medial side of the knee below the medial condyle of the tibia is an important area in acupuncture because passive acupoints can easily be found there in an overwhelming majority of people who have chronic pain from any cause. Five saphenous acupoints that are easily palpated are indicated in Figure 14.3a and Figure 14.3b.

The obturator nerve is another peripheral branch of the lumbar nerve plexus; it leaves the pelvis via the obturator foramen to supply skin and muscles in the medial compartment of the thigh. Several acupoints variably appear on the medial surface of the upper thigh. They are not often seen, except in cases of forceful abduction of the thigh, which might be sustained in a water skiing accident that damages the attachments of the hamstring muscles (semimembranosus and semitendinosus) to the pelvic bone.

### 14.2.2 THE SACRAL NERVE PLEXUS

The sacral nerve plexus (shown in Figure 14.4) is formed by the lumbosacral trunk and the anterior primary rami of the first three sacral spinal nerves. The lumbosacral trunk

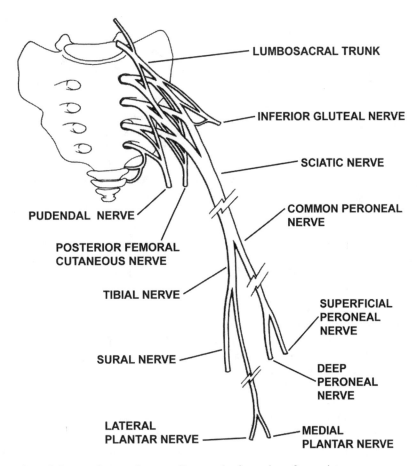

**FIGURE 14.4** The branches of the sacral nerve that contribute to the formation of acupoints.

consists of a portion of the anterior primary ramus of the fourth lumbar spinal nerve and the entire anterior primary ramus of the fifth lumbar spinal nerve. More than 20 different nerve branches come directly or indirectly from the sacral nerve plexus, although not all of them contribute to form the acupoints described later; those that do form acupoints are the inferior gluteal, the pudendal, the posterior femoral cutaneous, and the sciatic and its terminal branches. The sciatic nerve divides into two branches, the common peroneal and tibial; the common peroneal then subdivides into two terminal branches — the deep and superficial peroneals. The tibial nerve gives off a cutaneous branch known as the sural nerve in the posterior surface of the leg and also gives off the plantar nerves (lateral and medial) in the foot.

Branches of the sacral nerve plexus innervate skin and muscles of the gluteal region, posterior compartment of the thigh, popliteal fossa, posterior and lateral compartments of the leg, and muscles and skin of the entire foot. These nerves will be discussed next.

The inferior gluteal nerve arises from the posterior or dorsal branches of the anterior primary rami of the fifth lumbar and the first two sacral spinal nerves. It leaves the pelvis through the greater sciatic foramen below the piriformis muscle and enters the gluteus maximus muscle. This muscle is large and thick and the nerve deep within, yielding only one acupoint. This Inferior Gluteal (16) acupoint is located right in the center of the gluteal region, where the nerve enters the gluteus maximus muscle to form a neuromuscular attachment (see Figure 14.5). The location of the Inferior Gluteal acupoint has a rich vascular bed provided by the inferior gluteal artery and vein. Stubborn pain in the area of the point is sometimes referred to as piriformis muscle syndrome because of proximity of the nerve to the muscle and because the pain is purported to be produced by the muscle's clenching on the nerve. Such an explanation of the etiology of pain in the buttock is questionable for the simple reason that the piriformis is a small and deep muscle unlikely to be able to clench on the sciatic nerve. More likely, the pain originates from the acupoint formed by the neuromuscular attachment of the inferior gluteal nerve to the gluteus maximus muscle. The Inferior Gluteal point is important because it will appear tender in anyone who has low back pain.

The pudendal nerve is the major source of the rich innervation of the genitalia and anal sphincter. It controls defecation, facilitates penile erection, and affords protection to the testicles by the stimulation of muscular constrictions. Acupuncture may help some conditions resulting from a malfunction of this nerve; its acupoint is located lateral to the scrotum or labium majorus and was described in more detail in the previous chapter as the Pudendal point.

The posterior femoral cutaneous nerve branches from the sacral nerve plexus and emerges from the greater sciatic foramen distal to the piriformis muscle; it then descends under the gluteus maximus to reach the posterior surface of the thigh. Generally, this cutaneous nerve has two named branches relevant to this discussion. The first branch, often referred to as the gluteal branch, goes superiorly to the gluteal region as the recurrent nerve; it penetrates the gluteal fascia right at the center of the gluteal fold, forming the Gluteal Fold (U) acupoint. It innervates the lower buttocks and upper thigh. The second branch of the posterior femoral cutaneous nerve pierces the deep fascia at the middle of the central line of the posterior surface of the thigh, forming the Posterior Femoral Cutaneous (U) acupoint. This nerve innervates the middle and inferior areas of the posterior thigh.

The sciatic is the largest nerve trunk in the body and in most cadavers is finger-sized. In spite of its being the largest in diameter no acupoint can be attributed directly to this nerve because of its deep position. It divides into two terminal branches: the tibial and the common peroneal. A number of cutaneous branches of the sciatic nerve (usually four) can be traced directly from the sciatic nerve, but these are not acknowledged in texts and atlases of anatomy. These branches penetrate the iliotibial tract at the locations indicated in Figure 14.6. Because these nerves are not acknowledged or named in anatomical texts, the name "iliotibial" has been adopted to describe them. We believe these branches of the sciatic trunk are the cause of the condition known as meralgia paraesthetica, or pain along the lateral surface of the thigh; almost all of our low back pain patients complain of pain in this area and thus the acupoints formed by these branches are very important.

The common peroneal nerve arises from the lateral branch of the sciatic nerve. Pain originating from the sciatic nerve can course along the common peroneal nerve, even reaching to terminal branches of the superficial and deep peroneal nerves in the lateral compartment of the leg and the dorsal surface of the first three medial toes. Pain following this pattern is not uncommon in patients suffering from a long duration of chronic pain. (One uncommon source of pain in this nerve is hypodermic needle injections; the substance injected is more likely to cause injury than the needle.)

At the superior angle of the popliteal fossa, the common peroneal nerve follows the medial border of the biceps femoris muscle and its tendon following the superolateral boundary of the fossa, and then leaves the fossa by passing superficially to the lateral head of the gastrocnemius muscle. From there it passes over the back of the head of the fibula before winding around the lateral surface of the neck of the bone, finally running beneath the upper fibers of the peroneus longus muscle to enter the lateral muscular compartment of the leg. At the head of the fibula and posterolateral to its neck, the nerve can be palpated by rolling it against the bone. Here the nerve is very superficial, but no acupoint can be attributed to this loca-

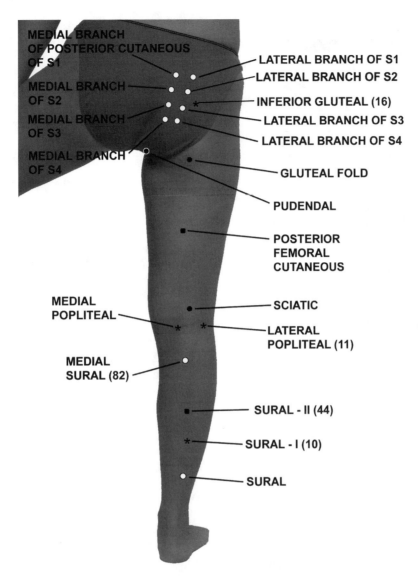

FIGURE 14.5 Acupoints from the sacral plexus in the gluteal region and on the posterior surface of the lower extremity.

tion, possibly because the nerve is still deep within the deep fascia without any branching or accompanying major blood vessels.

The common peroneal nerve bifurcates into the superficial and deep peroneal in the proximal region of the lateral compartment of the leg. The site of the bifurcation forms an important point, the Common Peroneal-I (24). Anatomically, the common peroneal and the deep radial in the forearm develop analogously in that, like the deep radial nerve with its multiple acupoints along its route, the common peroneal nerve has multiple points along its course as shown in Figure 14.7. As with the deep radial acupoints, the clinical significance of the Common Peroneal points diminishes distally.

The superficial and deep peroneal (called "fibular" by some authorities) are cutaneous nerves. The superficial peroneal surfaces above the deep fascia to innervate the skin of the dorsum of the foot, having pierced the fascia immediately lateral to the tendon of the extensor digitorum longus in the anterior ankle. At the site where the nerve pierces the fascia, the Superficial Peroneal (43) acupoint is formed. The superficial peroneal nerve distributes to the dorsum of the foot, forming a number of acupoints as shown in Figure 14.7. (The reader referring to an anatomical atlas while reading this text should be aware that these atlases contain many inaccuracies in depicting cutaneous nerves; this is particularly true of those of the feet.) The deep peroneal nerve becomes cutaneous approximately 2 cm rostral to the web between the great and second toes, forming the primary Deep Peroneal (5) acupoint. Nearly all patients seeking acupuncture treatment have sensitivity in this point.

The main trunk of the tibial nerve branches from the sciatic and remains in the posterior compartment of the

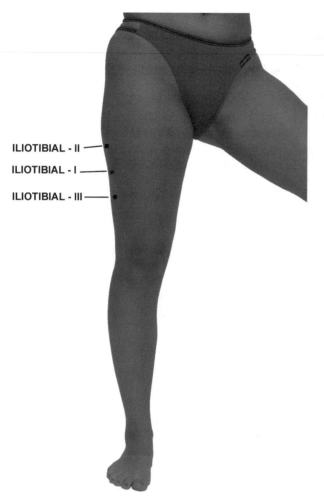

ILIOTIBIAL - II —

ILIOTIBIAL - I —

ILIOTIBIAL - III —

**FIGURE 14.6** The iliotibial acupoints.

leg, giving off muscular and cutaneous branches (Figure 14.8). The cutaneous branches contribute to the formation of Sural and Plantar acupoints, which are discussed later. The tibial nerve comes close to the skin about 7 to 8 cm above the medial malleolus, forming two named acupoints: the Tibial-I (6) and the Tibial-II (26), and often several nonspecific points as well. The skin surface over this area can become very sensitive in people with chronic pain and, as with the Deep Peroneal acupoint, nearly all patients seeking acupuncture treatment have tenderness over the Tibial-I acupoint. Distal to these points, the tibial nerve then courses into the foot and divides into two terminal branches, the medial and lateral plantar nerves (discussed later).

The sural nerve is actually formed by the union of the lateral sural branch from the common peroneal nerve and the medial sural branch from the tibial. These branches and the nerve they form contribute a primary, secondary, and nonspecific acupoint, the Sural-I (10), Sural-II (44), and Medial Sural (82), respectively (Figure 14.9). Other nonspecific acupoints can appear along these nerves in patients with pain in the posterior compartment of the leg.

Once the two branches come together to form the sural nerve, the nerve emerges from the deep fascia to become superficial on the posterior surface of the leg and then passes downward near the lateral margin of the calcaneus bone and Achilles tendon, supplying skin of the lateral and posterior aspects of the lower third of the leg. At the lateral margin of the tendon, the lateral Achilles (54) acupoint is formed.

The nerve continues below the lateral malleolus and along the lateral side of the foot and little toe, communicating on the dorsum of the foot with the superficial peroneal nerve. Many areas of the foot, particularly the lateral foot, have overlapping innervation between the sural and superficial peroneal nerves, and the acupoints that form in these areas are not easily assigned to either nerve branch (see Figure 14.10). These points are not often used in acupuncture, except in cases of local injury. They often become tender after the extremity has been splinted.

The medial and lateral plantar nerves are the terminal branches of the tibial nerve. The only named point formed by these two nerves is the Plantar (65), on the middle of the sole of the foot, but several other nonspecific points can form along their distribution. Sensory fibers are very dense on the soles of the feet, making them very tender to needles.

## 14.3  EXCEPTIONAL ACUPOINTS IN THE LOWER EXTREMITY

A few acupoints in the lower extremity are considered exceptional because, like the biceps tendon and the lateral epicondyle in the upper extremity, no discrete nerve element is associated with them. By far, the most important are the Medial and Lateral Popliteal points located in the popliteal fossa of the back of the knee. It was mentioned earlier (Chapter 4) that the medial acupoint is more important in young persons and the lateral acupoint becomes more important as the individual ages; only the Lateral Popliteal (11) is a numbered point. One of the popliteal points is always needled when a patient is treated in the prone position. The Lateral Popliteal point is located right next to the medial side of the tendon of the short head of the biceps femoris and the medial one is lateral to the tendons of the semitendinosus and semimembranosus muscles. No important cutaneous nerve is associated with either point. A branch of the posterior femoral cutaneous nerve is near, but not exactly at, the lateral point. The common peroneal nerve is deep below the lateral point and may have its division into the superficial and deep peroneal at this site.

Another important point is the Greater Trochanter (73), which is easily palpated on the side of the hip as a tubercle of the femur and is protected by a bursa. From one to six tender points can be palpated over the trochanter in patients with meralgia paraesthetica or trochanteric bur-

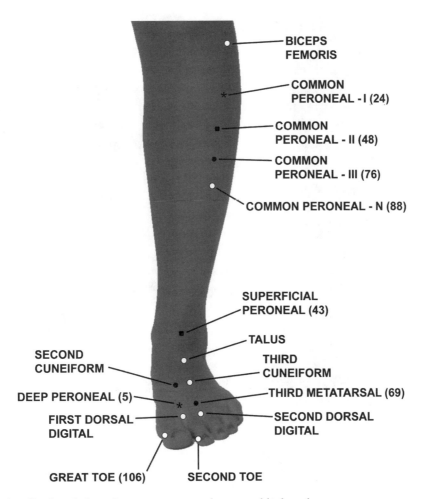

**FIGURE 14.7** Acupoints distributed along the common peroneal nerve and its branches.

sitis. The most likely cause of pain at the trochanter is inflammation of the bursa. The plantar surface of the calcaneus likewise has no discrete nerve element to form an acupoint, but occasionally becomes tender in one or several locations with a condition known as calcaneus fasciitis. This is a very tender location to place needles.

## 14.4 ACUPUNCTURE APPLIED TO CONDITIONS OF THE LOWER EXTREMITY

Painful conditions in the lower extremity affecting the hip and thigh, knee, leg, ankle, and foot will be discussed in the following paragraphs. The specific issue of phantom limb will be included in the discussion of the leg and that of peripheral neuropathy will be included with the foot.

### 14.4.1 CONDITIONS OF THE HIP AND THIGH

The anterior compartment of the thigh is innervated by the femoral nerve, which sends muscular branches to the quadriceps femoris and sartorius muscles and unnamed cutaneous branches to the sparsely innervated skin. Few

acupoints are over the anterior thigh and pain there is rare, typically seen only in crushing injuries. One example is Patsy, age 46, who sought acupuncture a few months after a severe motor vehicle accident for pain in both anterior thighs and also for sciatic pain on the right side. Both thighs had been crushed severely in the accident; she said that the entire anterior left thigh stayed blue for a couple of months. There were no fractures. Her left thigh was allodynic with pain perceived everywhere she was touched either deeply or lightly. Standing would aggravate the pain. Pain was also perceived on the right but it was less sensitive to touch. She said that the right thigh and leg were becoming worse because of favoring them in walking. Her pain was not quantified at the time but in retrospect it was probably about seven degrees.

Patsy's first treatment was done while she was in the supine position; primary points were needled along with a dozen points evenly spaced over the surface of the anterior compartment of each thigh. Two days later, she reported substantial improvement, having been able to stand without much problem the previous day; her thighs were still sensitive to touch. She was placed in the prone position and needles were placed in primary points and

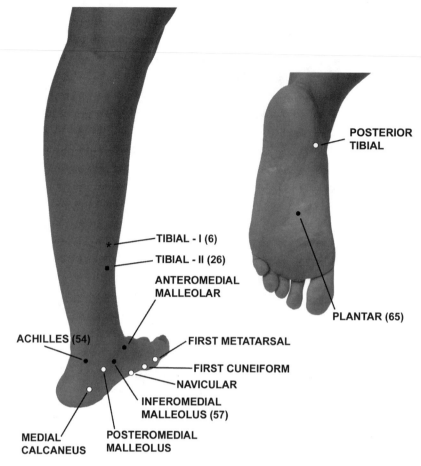

**FIGURE 14.8** Acupoints distributed along the tibial nerve and its branches.

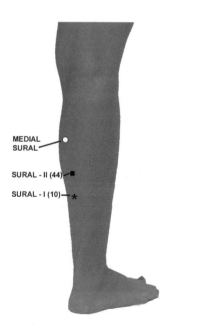

**FIGURE 14.9** Acupoints of the main branches of the sural nerve.

12 more were placed nonspecifically in each thigh — six along the lateral borders and six along the medial borders. By the third visit 2 days later, her back pain was resolved but she continued to have some pain in her left thigh. For eight more visits the treatment plan of the first two visits was repeated, alternating supine and prone positions. By then, the pain in her thighs had resolved, but she continued to come occasionally over the next 3 years when her back pain recurred. Patsy had 25 total acupuncture treatments.

The medial compartment contains gracilis and adductor muscles innervated by the well-protected obturator nerve. The muscles are occasionally injured, usually as a result of water skiing accidents, producing pain at their proximal ends near the inguinal region. This pain is usually easily treated with needles in the primary points and three or four needles in tender points in the affected area.

Pain in the posterior compartment (innervated by the sciatic nerve as described earlier) is not common except in some patients with long-standing back pain, who may describe a line of pain down the midline of the posterior thigh. Some may actually indicate the points where the nerves become cutaneous. Treatment consists of placing needles in the tender points.

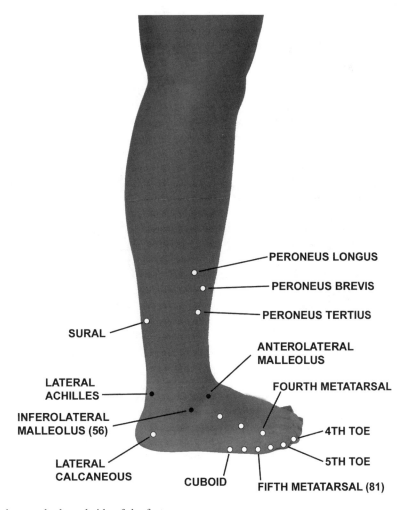

**FIGURE 14.10** Acupoints on the lateral side of the foot.

The enigma of meralgia paraesthetica was discussed previously. The nerve to which it is attributed by other authorities is essentially a nerve of the anterior compartment of the thigh, and the iliotibial tract where the pain of meralgia paraesthetica is perceived appears to be innervated by branches from the sciatic trunk. This is confirmed by the observation that patients with meralgia paraesthetica almost always have chronic low back pain, although other conditions such as arthritis and bursitis of the hip can produce the characteristic pain. Commonly, all three conditions — low back pain, meralgia paraesthetica, and pain over the greater trochanter — are seen together, suggesting a poorly understood relationship between trochanteric bursitis and meralgia paraesthetica.

Pain in the hip and lateral thigh is the second most commonly seen problem in the acupuncture clinic (after low back pain). It may be that inflammation of this bursa, the largest in the body , which is likely innervated by the sciatic nerve, irritates the nerve causing pain to be referred down the sciatic nerve to the branches seen to penetrate the iliotibial tract. Treatment for pain at the site of the bursa and along the lateral side of the thigh is similar to

that for low back pain described in the previous chapter, with the addition of the side position to place four to six needles into the bursa and four to six more in tender points along the iliotibial tract. Results are mixed; prior hip surgery generally suggests a poor prognosis.

## 14.4.2 CONDITIONS OF THE KNEE

Pain perceived as being in the knee can result from internal derangement of the joint, strains and sprains of structures around the joint, acupoints such as the Saphenous-I and the Common Peroneal-I that have transitioned to the active phase, and injuries of the back, hip, or ankle from which pain is referred to the knee. Several important acupoints around the knee are shown in Figure 14.11: the Saphenous-I (4); Lateral Popliteal (11); Common Peroneal-I (24); Femoral (31); Vastus Medialis (95); Vastus Lateralis (U); Medial and Lateral Parapatellar (U); and Biceps Femoris (U). (The Medial Popliteal, another important point, especially in young individuals, is not shown in the figure.)

Derangement within the joint includes worn out or torn cartilage, torn meniscus, fracture, arthritis, and disruption

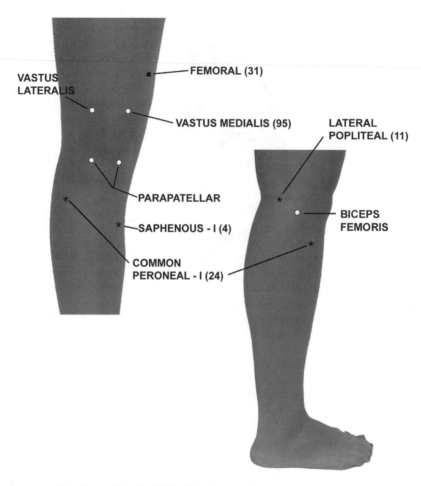

**FIGURE 14.11** Acupoints around the knee. The Medial Popliteal is not shown.

of the anterior or (rarely) the posterior cruciate ligaments. Internal derangement generally requires a surgical solution, but sometimes it is desirable to delay surgery or surgery is not possible or refused by the patient; in these instances, acupuncture can provide some degree of palliative relief. Tenderness along the medial or lateral joint lines (the Parapatellar acupoints on either side of the patellar tendon) is strongly suggestive of internal derangement, as is tenderness in the popliteal fossa medially or laterally. In treating osteoarthritis of the knee, a rule of thumb is that if only one of the two Parapatellar acupoints is tender, the knee will be easier to treat than if both are. Treatment for any of these conditions consists of placing needles in the points named previously and shown in Figure 14.11, plus those down the leg along the saphenous and common peroneal nerves, and of course the primary points.

Structures around the knee can also suffer sprains; most notably this affects the lateral collateral ligament or the medial collateral ligament. Injuries to these ligaments may accompany other injuries to the knee. These two ligaments respond quite readily to a few needles placed directly into them. The patella can become loose and track sloppily (most often to the lateral side), causing pain; this

is called the patellar–femoral syndrome and is thought to result from weakness in the quadriceps femoris muscle group. Many knee injuries can be avoided by strengthening these muscles and thus stabilizing the structure of the joint; physical therapy is a useful, even mandatory, adjunct to treating most causes of knee pain.

Another cause of pain perceived as coming from the knee is actually the transitioning of the Saphenous-I acupoint to the active state. Occasionally the Common Peroneal-I can become active and be perceived as pain within the knee. These acupoints may become active as a result of an acute knee injury that has since resolved; they may result from knee surgery; or they may be tender as part of a systemic response to pain elsewhere in the body. (As would be expected, knee surgery greatly complicates the acupuncture assessment of the joint.) Treatment consists of placing needles in the offending point and in other points along its nerve (these will almost certainly be passive) and in other passive points in the knee area. The prognosis depends primarily on the patient's pain sensitivity and the presence or absence of internal knee derangement.

Finally, knee pain may accompany sciatica or meralgia paraesthetica, or may even result from a hip or ankle injury; in the presence of knee pain, it is important to assess the joints above and below the painful joint. Treatment consists of treating the source of the pain along with any passive acupoints in the region of the knee.

### 14.4.3 Conditions in the Leg

In the calf, burning, tingling, and numbness superficially or cramping with deep aching most likely come from the sural nerves — cutaneous nerves which run deep inside the deep fascia of the legs. Although claudication, a condition caused by ischemia of the leg muscles due to sclerosis with narrowing of the arteries, must be ruled out by arterial studies (e.g., ultrasound), many of these patients have normal arterial flow. Their pain is easily managed with three sessions, repeated occasionally as needed depending on their pain quantification. Primary points are needled with 6 to 12 additional needles placed nonspecifically around the painful calf area.

On the front surface of the leg, pain in the shin is associated with the common peroneal distribution; in teenagers it is called "growing pains" and is easy to manage. The condition in adults is much more difficult to treat. The treatment is the same for either group, however: a few needles are placed in a row a couple of centimeters lateral to the lateral margin of the tibia along its length, starting with the Common Peroneal-I acupoint, and continuing from passive point to passive point. Needles should be placed in any tender primary or secondary points systemically, but in a teenager of low pain sensitivity, it may be adequate simply to place needles along the tibia. Pain on the lateral side of the leg in the area of the peroneus longus and brevis muscles also comes from the peroneal distribution; this pain is not too common, but is easily treated with needles along the tibia as just described and additional needles placed nonspecifically where pain is perceived.

Another issue in the leg is phantom limb pain seen after an amputation. Phantom limb is a controversial medical issue with some authorities debating its existence.[5-7] According to Bonica, "the role of preamputation pain in the genesis of phantom limb pain is unclear. Some have suggested that pain prior to amputation increases the likelihood of severe phantom limb pain. Others have not found this association."[8] We have seen eight cases of phantom limb so far, all involving the lower extremity. All of the patients were quantified to have pain at seven degrees or higher, up to ten. Pain at these sensitivities is difficult to manage, phantom or otherwise. At best, we have had temporary success requiring frequent repeated treatments.

### 14.4.4 Conditions in the Ankle

Ankle sprains are quite common, affecting ligaments connecting the tibia, fibula, calcaneus, and talus. Most are self-limited, but in some cases ligaments can be torn to the extent that they require surgical correction. Even if the ligaments are intact, however, pain can cause favoring the opposite extremity and concomitant weakness of the musculature around the affected ankle. Caught early while the pain is acute, this condition is easily treated with needles, reducing morbidity and the need for extensive therapy for lower grade sprains. Usually, all that is needed is needles in the Inferolateral Malleolar (56) and Inferomedial Malleolar (57) acupoints; and in any other tender ligaments in the ankle and other tender primary points throughout the body. It should be remembered that pain in the ankle may come from the back, hip, or knee, so these causes should be sought. Higher degree patients with chronic pain may be refractory to acupuncture management, but acute cases generally respond well.

### 14.4.5 Conditions in the Foot

Pain in the feet not resulting from peripheral neuropathy is generally treated by needling systemic points and painful points in the feet. Causes may be bunions or neuromas (e.g., Morton's neuroma) or acute contusions or sprains. Bunions, most often seen on the medial side of the big toes and occasionally on the lateral side of the little toes, unilaterally or bilaterally, are easy to treat. Pain is usually limited to the affected toe, but may extend to either side of the foot posteriorly to the heel and under the plantar surface. Pain involving a more extensive area of the foot understandably has a more complicated etiology and will be harder to deal with than pain limited to the area of bunions alone. The skin of bunions often appears erythyemic but may be of normal appearance. A few needles placed nonspecifically into the bunion and other passive points in the foot, along with primary points throughout the body, should suffice, although if the patient continues to wear pointed or tight shoes the bunion will continue to grow.

Another condition of the foot is called "Morton's neuroma," although surgically no neuroma can be found in many, if not most, patients. It presents as pain on the dorsum of the foot in the web spaces, usually between the third and fourth toes, but occasionally between the fourth and fifth or second and third. In the early stages, the condition is easily treated with needles in the web spaces where pain is perceived. Similarly, pain on the bottom of the foot (plantar fasciitis, tarsal tunnel syndrome) is usually easily treated, although noncompliance is a problem because of the sensitivity of the area. Pain in the heel can be relieved with a needle into the Calcaneus acupoint; pain in the center of the foot can be relieved with a needle in the Plantar acupoint; and that between adjacent metatarsal heads can be relieved with a needle in the tender spot where pain is perceived. Pain on the bottom of the foot almost always requires three treatments even though patients will often claim that pain is completely gone after the first treatment. Pain in a toe can usually be relieved with one needle on each side of the affected digit.

Peripheral neuropathy deserves special mention. Peripheral neuropathy can affect motor or sensory nerves, or both. Patients with motor nerve problems are not often seen in the acupuncture clinic and are rarely helped. Most patients have problems related to sensory nerve malfunctions, such as pain, cold, burning, pricking, stinging, stabbing, and numbing sensations; most suffer a combination of these sensations, but rarely all of them. Generally, pain is the easiest sensation to control and numbness the most difficult (it is thought that the nerve fibers carrying sensations of numbness are larger than those carrying pain).

Successful management depends on low pain sensitivity and relatively low duration of symptoms; the specific etiology, such as diabetes, alcoholism, toxic exposures, radiotherapy, chemotherapy, or trauma, is less predictive of success. Neuropathy from chronic causes tends to begin at the big toe and extend to the other toes, up the foot and into the leg. If it is caught before it extends past the ankle, it is fairly easily managed, but once it extends to the knees, acupuncture has no effect. In one case, a patient with only three degrees of pain sensitivity but also with continuing kidney failure relapsed repeatedly over nearly 200 treatments, suggesting that the cause must be removed to attain permanent benefit. Treatment of peripheral neuropathy consists of placing needles in primary points and around the margins of the affected area.

## REFERENCES

1. Dung, H.C. Acupuncture points of the lumbar plexus. *Am. J. Chin. Med.* 13:133, 1985.
2. Dung, H.C. Acupuncture points of the sacral plexus. *Am. J. Chin. Med.* 13:145, 1985.
3. Hollinshead, W.H. *Anatomy for Surgeons,* Vol. 3. *Back and Limbs.* Harper and Row, New York, 1969. See also Moore, K.L. *Clinical Oriented Anatomy.* Williams and Wilkins, Baltimore, 1980; Warwich, R. and Williams, P.L. *Gray's Anatomy.* W.B. Saunders, Philadelphia, 1984; Woodburne, R.T. *Essentials of Human Anatomy,* 8th ed. Oxford University Press, New York, 1988.
4. See, for example, Asimov, I. et al. *Stedman's Medical Dictionary,* 21st ed. Williams and Wilkins, Baltimore, 971, 1966.
5. Kelley, W.N. et al. *Textbook of Rheumatology,* Vols. I and II. W.B. Saunders Company, Philadelphia, 1993.
6. Sherman, R.A. and Sherman, C.J. Prevalence and characteristics of chronic phantom limb pain among American veterans. *Am. J. Phys. Med.* 62:227, 1983.
7. Kegel, B. et al. A surgery of lower-limb amputee: prostheses, phantom sensations, and psychosocial aspects. *Bull. Prosth. Res.* 114:43, 1977.
8. Bonica, J.J. *The Management of Pain,* 2nd ed. Vol. I and II. Lea & Febiger, Philadelphia, 1990.

# 15 Other Considerations

## CONTENTS

A few issues have been left unresolved in this text. One concerns uses of acupuncture not previously mentioned; another deals with areas of future research and yet another concerns the practical aspects of including acupuncture in a medical practice. These are discussed in this chapter.

## 15.1 OTHER CONDITIONS

There are a number of other conditions in which we have tried to use acupuncture (mostly with limited results) and possibly others we have overlooked. Regarding the latter, we look forward to seeing innovative studies of our peers in the medical literature. Regarding the former, a few deserve mention:

- Hiatal hernia pain can often be relieved with two to four needles around the xiphoid process of the sternum (T5 dermatome).
- Gall bladder disease can be ameliorated with a couple of needles under the costal arch (T6).
- Ulcerative colitis and irritable bowel syndrome are generally unresponsive, although minor irritation of the gastrointestinal tract can be relieved by needling the primary points and thus increasing parasympathetic stimulation and intestinal motility.
- For psoriasis and psoriatic arthritis, acupuncture offers no relief.
- For connective tissue disorders, acupuncture is occasionally palliative.
- Itching skin occasionally responds to needles quite well.
- Erythema multiforme had gratifying results in our only case.
- For multiple sclerosis, acupuncture is useless, as it is also for lupus erythematosus.

- Reflex sympathetic dystrophy may show positive response to needles placed in the primary points and around the margins of the painful area and any painful scars.
- For so-called chronic fatigue syndrome, acupuncture has not shown any benefit.

Some of these conditions affecting the gastrointestinal tract were discussed briefly in Chapter 13; the issues of arthritis and osteoporosis deserve special mention.

Rheumatoid arthritis is a chronic systemic disease, thought to have an autoimmune etiology, that primarily affects the joints. As a chronic disease, it typically progresses subclinically for years before being diagnosed. Once rheumatoid arthritis is diagnosed, the patient is prescribed nonsteroidal anti-inflammatory drugs (NSAIDs); as the disease progresses, other drugs are tried and, ultimately, the patient may end up on steroids. In advanced stages of the disease, the proximal interphalangeal joints of the hands and feet and other joints may become deformed. By this time, the patient will typically have high pain sensitivity and the disease will be refractory to treatment. The existence of deformity of the joints is a bad prognostic sign because needles will not restore a structural abnormality and the deformed structure is a likely cause of pain in addition to the pain of inflammation. Generally, patients come for acupuncture in an advanced stage of the disease and obtain limited results. Two more fortunate patients are described next.

Nancy, a 43-year-old woman, demonstrates that rheumatoid arthritis pain can be managed with acupuncture in some individuals. She was assessed at eight degrees when she first presented at the clinic. She was taking daily steroids and had the characteristic "moon face." She complained of pain in the proximal interphalangeal joints of her fingers, especially the middle and ring fingers of both hands, and in her left knee; she had less severe pain in the right knee as well. She said the pain was continuous, sometimes waxing or waning, but never relieved.

During her first two visits, she was needled in primary points only — the first visit supine and the second prone. When she came for the third visit, she did not seem to have had any flare-up of pain from the needles, so she was placed in a sitting position and needles were placed in primary and secondary points, as well as tertiary and non-specific points, on the dorsum of each hand; both sides of the proximal interphalangeal joints of the middle three fingers; and both knees, with an emphasis on the left, where a total of 12 needles was placed around the knee joint.

When she came for her fourth visit 2 days later, it appeared that she was having a flare-up from the needles of the third visit because her left knee was considerably more painful. She was placed in a prone position; needles were placed in the primary points and three additional needles were placed in each popliteal fossa plus three more along the saphenous nerve points. She then had three more treatment sessions repeating the plan of the first three visits. When she came for her seventh visit, she had had some fluid withdrawn from her left knee and received a steroid injection; at that time, her pain was greatly diminished. She continued to have three more treatments; after those she was practically pain free everywhere. We recommended that she return for three more visits a month later, but she did not heed that recommendation. She was encountered socially about 8 months later and said that her pain had not returned. Of course, it is not known what affect the steroid injection had on her improvement.

Louis, a 60-year-old male, is another example. He had been diagnosed with rheumatoid arthritis 2 years previously and was taking prednisone and ibuprofen to manage his arthritis pain, but was beginning to have gastrointestinal irritation from the medications. His pain sensitivity was estimated to be five degrees, although he had many passive points around his shoulder and knee joints. The first treatment was administered with Louis in the supine position, using the primary points with the addition of three needles along each biceps brachii tendon in the shoulders. On his second visit, he reported less pain and better sleep; he was treated in the prone position with needles in the primary points only. He was substantially improved on his third visit and was treated in the supine position with additional needles in the dorsum of each wrist. He came for his fourth visit 2 days later and said he had been pain free for about a day. He was then treated in the prone position by apparently using only the primary points (the record is unclear on this point).

On his fifth visit, his pain had flared up, possibly caused by his sitting in a room that was too cold while attending a conference the day before. On that visit, he was placed in the sitting position, with a number of primary and secondary points needled, along with eight needles in each knee and shoulder. On the sixth visit, he said

the pain had diminished again. He went on to have five more treatments over the next month and was then pain free. Two months later, the pain had returned and Louis came in for two more treatments. Thereafter, he would come every 3 or 4 months for four or fewer treatments. As time went on, the pain recurred less frequently, such that the 29th treatment gave him 3 years of relief and the 30th treatment gave him 6 years of relief, after which he returned for five more treatments. He had been successfully managed with 35 treatments over a 10-year period.

Osteoporosis is another systemic disease, affecting primarily females; it is a complex and poorly understood disorder of metabolism resulting in demineralization of bones. It does not usually cause pain in itself, but as the bones weaken, they may spontaneously fracture, becoming a source of chronic pain. Women seeking help in the acupuncture clinic typically are over 65 years of age, not overweight, and have a somewhat increased kyphosis in the thoracic spine. They typically describe their pain as being in the area of the intrinsic back muscles of the erector spinae in the dermatomes from T6 to T12. On palpation, tender points can usually be appreciated 2 or 3 cm lateral to the mid-sagittal line in these dermatomes. These are the points at which the muscular branch of the posterior primary ramus of each thoracic spinal nerve makes its attachment. Needles should be placed in these points and as many tender primary and secondary points as practical. These are typically individuals with high pain sensitivity, so multiple treatment sessions and frequent relapses are likely.

Mentioned several times previously in this text, fibromyalgia is considered to be a disease of the connective tissue and is thought to have a systematic cause. Patients with the disease complain of pain in many areas of the body. Some experts question the existence of the disease altogether. Interestingly enough, fibromyalgia was mentioned in medical publications more than half a century ago. By the 1980s, a resurgence of interest in the disease had occurred, but that did not greatly increase understanding of it[1-5] and the subject is still controversial. Further complicating the issue is the fact that these patients may complain of pain anywhere in the body: some have headache; some have pain in the upper limbs; and some have pain in the low back. These patients often express that their treating physicians do not seem to take their complaints seriously and cannot tell them what is wrong.

Before 1990, not many patients had been diagnosed with fibromyalgia, but now it is a common diagnosis. A number of authorities have defined this condition as tenderness in a certain percentage of defined sites on the body. These sites are almost invariably those defined in this text as primary acupoints. According to these definitions, a large majority of patients in our acupuncture clinic could be diagnosed with fibromyalgia. If they only had those primary points tender to palpation, they would have low pain sensitivities and thus be easy to manage; thus it can be seen that this type of definition leads to a test that is too sensitive. In reality, when patients tell us that their doctors have diagnosed them as having fibromyalgia, we find the patients to have pain sensitivities of seven degrees or higher. These patients are definitely difficult to manage, as we have shown throughout this text. Pain diagnosed as fibromyalgia is easy to treat, usually in three or four treatments, for patients quantified to have a pain level of four or fewer degrees. Pain becomes harder to manage when the level goes up to five to eight degrees. Once pain exceeds nine degrees, acupuncture will not likely be useful.

Conceptually, we treat fibromyalgia patients the same as we would any other chronic pain patient. (We are not convinced of any difference, other than terminology, in the two types of patients.) The first two treatments are limited to primary points administered in varying positions to allow access to as many points as possible. Starting with the third treatment, more needles can be added; a general guideline for increasing the number of needles to be used is to add incrementally 8 to 10 each time, up to a maximum of about 50 (occasionally as many as 60). The additional needles are placed in the tenderest acupoints in the general area or areas in which the patient perceives pain.

## 15.2 FUTURE RESEARCH

The conditions described above are mostly questionable or marginal uses of acupuncture, in which its role needs further definition and understanding and is awaiting further research. Other areas of potential research have been mentioned throughout this text, and it may be fruitful to reiterate them here. Hopefully, bright minds will be challenged by the twin enigmas of pain and acupuncture and by some of the other issues that this book has broached.

First and foremost, Dung's original research should be repeated, and the points listed in this book as "unnumbered" should be included in that research. Parallel research should be done on "normal" individuals randomly selected from the general population ("normal" meaning those without pain complaints). Dung's original research suffers in that he determined the tender points, administered treatment, and measured outcomes himself; it should be repeated in an environment in which one person measures sensitivity, another provides treatment, and yet another measures outcome (or the patient could do so on an analog scale). Each of the experimenters should be blind to the others' work. Although this does not meet the standards of a randomly controlled trial, it at least greatly reduces the possibility of observer bias in testing the null hypothesis that pain sensitivity does not affect outcome. Surely, other researchers will think of more rigorous ways to test our basic tenets of pain sensitivity; we hope that some will take sufficient notice of the huge problem of

pain and the potential benefits of measuring pain sensitivity to put our ideas to the most rigorous testing.

A related area of research would be to follow a cohort of individuals over time, recording and correlating each one's pain sensitivity; blood pressure; menstrual history (if applicable); and pain complaints (quantified on an analog scale), including particularly neck and shoulder pain, back pain, TMJ, migraine headache, and carpal tunnel syndrome. It would be useful in our understanding of the development of chronic pain to record these variables at least annually from ages 10 to 20 and every 5 years thereafter. These individuals should be further tested to provide clues as to whether certain psychological traits make some more prone to rapidly increasing pain sensitivities. Does depression or anxiety affect pain sensitivity? Another question that should be answered is the effect of certain chronic diseases, e.g., diabetes, on sensitivity. Yet another is whether pain sensitivity affects the severity or nature of menopausal symptoms. Another area of research would be to measure pain sensitivities to see if they change through the menstrual cycle.

We have mentioned earlier in this text that acupuncture works for some conditions but the duration of action is uncertain. Hypertension is one such area. It would be helpful to know if response is sufficiently predictable to allow acupuncture to be used as a treatment for this problem. Perhaps in the future a wearable device, somewhat similar to a TENS unit, that stimulates the peripheral nervous system and controls blood pressure could be developed; this could significantly increase compliance and reduce the cost of treating this important disease. We have had success using acupuncture for urinary incontinence; does this suggest future treatments utilizing specific nerve stimulation? Surely these are speculative musings, but they are offered to show how little we know about the potential of controlling the peripheral nervous system and, indirectly, visceral organs. The opportunities for research in this area are boundless; the effects and their duration need to be quantified and a theoretical model needs to be developed to explain them.

It would be helpful to have a better understanding of the chemical changes within peripheral nerves of organisms exposed to chronic pain. Another area of research would be to determine changes that occur in nerve conduction velocities in individuals as their pain sensitivities increase. Chapter 2 discussed two models to describe the progression of passive acupoints: one based on anatomical features and another on the mechanical affect on a nerve from palpating it with a fixed amount of pressure. These two models should be compared because, if the difference in pain sensitivities turns out to be a function of effective palpation pressure (measured as the pressure per unit area on the surface of the nerve) rather than of any specific characteristics of individual nerves, that would suggest that pain perceived anywhere in the body causes permanent chemical changes throughout the peripheral nervous system. If these chemical changes were to be understood, it might be possible to reverse them chemically.

A related question — an important one not addressed throughout this text — is the mechanism of acupuncture's effect: how does it work? We do not feel that we have enough knowledge to answer this question. We know that it increases the endorphin level in the brain, although we suspect that this is not a direct effect, and further that it causes release of norepinephrine from postganglionic sympathetic fibers, possibly exhausting the supply of that neurotransmitter. We know that acupuncture is a strong suppressor of sympathetic tone and enhances parasympathetic tone. Also, it may be that the release of norepinephrine during needling suppresses prostaglandin, which would account for the decrease in cramping that is frequently seen.

Another neurotransmitter involved in acupuncture is histamine, which produces the characteristic atopic skin reaction shown in Figure 8.5; this reaction is significantly stronger in the Paravertebral points located along the thoracic sympathetic trunk. The histamine is likely released from mast cells in reaction to needle stimulation, dilating smooth muscle in nearby blood vessels and producing the atopic reaction. In short, the most we know about acupuncture's mechanism of action is how little we know. We applaud earlier work by Pomeranz and others cited in the appendix of this text and hope that a new generation of researchers will continue and expand this pioneering work. We hope to be able to report new and exciting discoveries about acupuncture's mechanism of action in the next edition of this text.

## 15.3   PRACTICAL ASPECTS

The future of medical acupuncture lies in the primary care specialties. We have repeatedly touted the benefits of early acupuncture intervention, and it is mainly primary care practitioners who can offer its benefits soon enough to make a difference. Certainly applications exist in other specialties:

- Cancer chemotherapists will find it very helpful to control nausea, vomiting, and pain.
- Allergists, otolaryngologists, and pulmonologists will find its effects on the sinuses and lungs to be an important adjunct to (or replacement for) pharmacologic treatment.
- Interventional radiologists will use needles to treat the important complication of xerostomia.
- Ophthalmologists will find it helpful to treat dry eye conditions.

Undoubtedly, applications in many specialties have not even crossed our minds; however, the basic use of acupuncture is in primary care. Recognizing this reality, we want to share some of the more practical aspects of using acupuncture in one's practice.

First, though, one obvious aspect needs to be discussed: education. Medical education is difficult, in that many students arrive idealistic and enthusiastic to treat patients only to be confronted with two difficult years of basic sciences before they are really allowed to initiate treatment with any patient. (Of course, some medical schools have tinkered with this problem, but the basic problem remains that students need to have some knowledge before they start treating patients.) By this time, many students have been discouraged or hardened by the rigorous demands of their first 2 years, which, for most curricula, lack real clinical relevance to students. This is a basic problem of medical education that acupuncture can help solve. One of the potentially most tedious and noxious subjects in those first 2 years is gross anatomy: dissection is messy and stinky and the detail is unending. Using an anatomical approach, acupuncture can make the discipline much more acceptable to beginning students, to whom it can be taught early in their education with a minimum of risk to any patient. They can treat each other or real patients and acupuncture can bring the study of anatomy to life. Furthermore, acupuncture is really so easy to perform and the results so gratifying that students can easily get a real taste of the rewards of medicine early in their careers.

Licensed practitioners who have not been taught acupuncture should still have the opportunity to learn. Time, money, complexity, and licensing issues are among the perceived barriers to learning acupuncture. Actually, time is rarely an issue because a weekend course is sufficient to teach the basic knowledge and skills, especially if the practitioner can undertake a little advance study — this text has been designed to be helpful in this regard. The cost of such a course should be within the budget of most practices, especially considering the financial benefits addressed in the following paragraph. To one who understands basic anatomy or who is willing to undertake a brief review of the subject, acupuncture is not complex but really quite simple: needle the primary points and a few additional tender ones in the area where pain is perceived; add a few secondary points where necessary.

Licensing issues are thornier because in some states legislators have been convinced by practitioners of oriental medicine that it is necessary to learn an arcane system of meridians and herbs to be able to stick needles into patients. This is ridiculous: sticking needles into patients to do trigger point injections of drugs can be done with impunity, but in some states, if the needles carry no drugs, the law has been violated. If oriental medicine practitioners have the clout to convince their states that they should be able to stick needles into people without any knowledge of scientific medical concepts, then their use of acupuncture becomes an issue between themselves and their patients. However, for states to declare that licensed medical doctors cannot practice the skills described in this text has absolutely no basis. Perhaps, in those states, practitioners can finesse these issues by recasting acupuncture as neuromodulation, as described in Chapter 1.

One of the most frequently asked questions from practitioners is whether or not insurers will pay for acupuncture. Although most do, many do not. Again, recasting the procedure as neuromodulation may help. Hopefully, the academic underpinning provided by this text can provide additional ammunition for the practitioner trying to get paid for his or her work. However, even if the insurer will not pay for acupuncture, it almost always pays for the office visit, and that may be sufficient given that the time required to place needles is so short (3 to 5 minutes). One of the major constraints to incorporating acupuncture into a practice is space: an acupuncture patient ties up a room for 20 to 25 minutes, and if rooms are in short supply, this can seriously slow down a busy practice. Another consideration in inaugurating acupuncture into a practice is the necessity to train personnel adequately in the proper handling of the patient and the needles, especially if the needles are to be recycled.

A final word is in order for those considering adding acupuncture to their practices. In the preface to this text, one of the authors' wavering prior to undertaking the study of acupuncture was mentioned. Those words should be reviewed — the gratification a practitioner feels when a patient responds dramatically to a procedure as simple, quick, and time-honored as acupuncture cannot be described. It is so easy to learn and to incorporate into one's practice that there is no reason not to undertake it.

## REFERENCES

1. Smythe, H. Tender points: evolution of concepts of the fibrositis/fibromyalgia syndrome. *Am. J. Med.* 81:3, 1986.
2. Yunus, M.B. Diagnosis, etiology, and management of fibromyalgia syndrome. An update. *Compr. Ther.*, 14:8, 1988.
3. Simms, R.W. et al. Tenderness in 71 anatomic sites: distinguishing fibromyalgia patients from controls. *Arthritis Rheum.* 31:182, 1988.
4. Goldenberg, D.L. Fibromyalgia syndrome. *JAMA* 257:1782, 1987.
5. Wolfe, F. et al. The American College of Rheumatology 1990 criteria for the classification of fibromyalgia: report of the Multicenter Criteria Committee. *Arthritis Rheum.* 33:160, 1990.

# Appendix

## Review of Neuroanatomy as Applied to Acupuncture

## CONTENTS

## A.1 DIVISIONS OF THE NERVOUS SYSTEM

Anatomically, the nervous system is described as being divided into the central and the peripheral nervous systems. The peripheral nervous system (PNS) is an extension of the central nervous system (CNS).

### A.1.1 THE CENTRAL NERVOUS SYSTEM

The *central nervous system* (CNS) consists of the brain and spinal cord. The brain is housed in the skull or cranial bones and the spinal cord in the vertebral canal. Despite a few reports published by Pomeranz,[1–4] Pert,[5] Wenhe,[6,7] and Ulett,[8] the response of the brain and spinal cord to acupuncture stimulation is poorly understood.

### A.1.2 THE PERIPHERAL NERVOUS SYSTEM

The *peripheral nervous system* (PNS) is all neural tissue or structure outside the brain and spinal cord. It is the most important anatomical element relating to an under-standing of acupuncture. If needles reduce pain, it must be because they interact with pain fibers of the PNS.

It is helpful to keep in mind that the PNS is the extension of the central nervous system and is entirely composed of nerve fibers originating in the 12 cranial nerves of the brain and the 33 pairs of spinal nerves of the spinal cord. The 12 cranial nerves are: olfactory (I); optic (II); oculomotor (III); trochlear (IV); trigeminal (V); abducens (VI); facial (VII); vestibulocochlear, also known as statoacoustic (VIII); glossopharyngeal (IX); vagus (X); spinal accessory (XI); and hypoglossal (XII).

Not all cranial nerves are relevant to acupuncture. The most important is the trigeminal (V), followed by the facial (VII) and the spinal accessory (XI). The vestibulo-cochlear (VIII), glossopharyngeal (IX), and vagus (X) nerves are only occasionally relevant.

The 33 pairs of spinal nerves are grouped into 8 cervical pairs, 12 thoracic, 5 lumbar, 5 sacral, and 3 coccygeal pairs, corresponding to the level of their emergence from the spinal cord.

0-8493-1651-0/04/$0.00+$1.50
© 2004 by CRC Press LLC

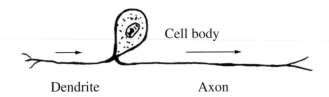

**FIGURE A.1** A bipolar (sensory) neuron. Information flows from dendrite to cell body to axon.

The *nerve fibers* in the PNS are distributed to nearly all areas of the body. A nerve fiber is a portion of a nerve cell ("neuron").

## A.2 NEURONS

Neurons, as nerve cells are called, are the structural units of the nervous system. They are classified according to their morphology (i.e., unipolar, bipolar, or multipolar); their location (e.g., pyramidal neuron, Purkinje neuron of the cerebellum, ventral horn neuron); and their function (i.e., motor neurons, sensory neurons, or neurons of the sympathetic or parasympathetic ganglia). The main focus in this text is the bipolar (sensory) neuron. See Figure A.1 for a depiction of a typical bipolar neuron. The cell body of a bipolar neuron is housed in a structure known as a *ganglion*. These ganglia are found outside the central nervous system. In the case of the cranial nerves, two important ganglia are the trigeminal, which belongs to the trigeminal nerve, and the pterygopalatine, which belongs to the facial nerve. The trigeminal ganglion is also known as the semilunar ganglion because it looks like a half moon. For each of the 33 pairs of spinal nerves, ganglia are situated just beside the spinal cord that are called *dorsal root ganglia* (also known as *spinal ganglia*) because of their location on the dorsal root of each of the spinal nerves (Figure A.2).

A neuron basically consists of a cell body, a dendrite or dendrites, and an axon (Figure A.1). A multipolar neuron may have several dendrites but the bipolar sensory neurons that are of more concern in this text have only one. Dendrites and axons are protoplasmic processes extending from the cell body and comprise the *nerve fibers*, or *nerves*. Cell bodies, dendrites, and axons of neurons are situated in a framework of specialized connective or interstitial tissue known as *neuroglia*.

## A.3 NERVE FIBERS

All biologic or physiologic messages are transmitted through nerves, much as electrical information is transmitted through wire (or, alternatively, messages may be transmitted by circulating hormones). Biologic information moving through nerves proceeds in only one direction, from dendrite to cell body to axon (Figure A.1), where it may then communicate with another nerve or adjacent tissue. The nerve fibers that carry messages away from the CNS are known as efferent (or motor) fibers and are all axons. Acupuncture is of very little use in dealing with diseases of efferent nerves, particularly those to voluntary skeletal muscles. This text will cover mostly afferent (or sensory) fibers — dendrites that conduct messages or information toward the CNS. It is helpful to keep in mind that *afferent* and *sensory* are two different names for the dendrites of sensory neurons.

This understanding of the direction of information flow in nerves suggests a powerful fact: acupuncture has little use in treating diseases of the motor nerves. All cell bodies of motor nerves are housed in the central nervous system. Nerve impulses generated in the motor nerve cells are carried outward to the peripheral areas of the body by way of efferent fibers. Any messages created by needle stimulation of the peripheral nervous system along any efferent fibers cannot be reversed to reach back to the

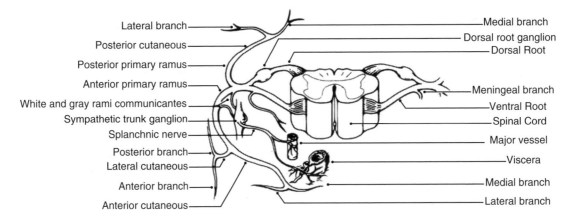

**FIGURE A.2** A typical spinal nerve and the dorsal root ganglia. Each of the six terminal cutaneous branches of the spinal nerve represents an acupoint around a dermatome. A sympathetic ganglion and its connections from the spinal cord to adjacent levels to form the sympathetic chain and to visceral organs through the splanchnic nerve.

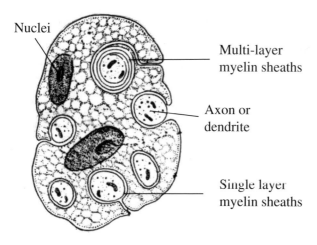

**FIGURE A.3** The formation of myelin sheaths around six axons or dendrites. Most of the fibers have only a single layer of myelin but one is shown with three layers. Two neuroglia cell ("Schwann cell") nuclei are shown.

motor cell bodies. Therefore, acupuncture essentially works through sensory nerves — afferent dendritic fibers that carry impulses back to the CNS.

Like electrical wires, nerve fibers carry electrical impulses and, to keep from "shorting out," they must be insulated. The material used to insulate nerve fibers is *myelin*, a sheath consisting of lipid (fat) formed by cells in the neuroglia that is an ideal biological insulation for nerves. Figure A.3 depicts a small bundle of nerve fibers cut cross sectionally to show axons and dendrites with their myelin sheaths in a small bundle. As can be seen from the figure, axons and dendrites are rather uniform in size as protoplasmic or cytoplasmic extensions of the nerve cell bodies. The main factor contributing to variations of the nerve fiber size is the thickness of the myelin sheaths surrounding them. Some nerves may not have much myelin wrapping; these are referred to as "unmyelinated fibers." The diameter of nerves in a cross section can differ by a magnitude of 10 or more, depending on how much myelin surrounds the nerve fibers. Nerve fibers are structurally or anatomically categorized according to their sizes, and different sizes of nerves often have different physiologic functions. For example, efferent fibers are likely to be larger because they generally have more myelin covering.

# A.4 CATEGORIZATION OF PERIPHERAL NERVE FIBERS

The following categorization of peripheral nerves is typical. Although the information is complex, the portion directly relevant to acupuncture is the discussion of afferent fibers for the general senses, postganglionic sympathetic nerve fibers, and efferent fibers to the skeletal muscles. The postganglionic sympathetic nerve fibers are discussed later in this appendix.

## A.4.1 AFFERENT FIBERS

Sensation in the body originates from sensory receptors and is transmitted to the CNS by afferent fibers. It is important to note that sensation can also be created and produced along any segment of these afferent fibers, not just at the terminal receptors. This is essential to understanding acupuncture because the needles are able to stimulate not only sensory receptors but also the afferent nerve fibers. Histologically, sensory nerves belong to two major categories: those for the special senses and those for the general senses.

### A.4.1.1 For Special Senses

The term *special senses* is used histologically to indicate that each is located in a special area (all are in the head) and each has a unique physiologic duty to perform. The five special senses are

1. Smell (olfactory; from receptors in the olfactory epithelium in the upper portion of the nose to cranial nerve I)
2. Vision (optic; from the retina of each eye to cranial nerve II)
3. Taste (facial; from taste buds on the tongue to cranial nerve VII)
4,5. Hearing and equilibrium (vestibulocochlear or statoacoustic; from the inner ear within the temporal bone to cranial nerve VIII). The receptors for hearing in the inner ear are in a structure known as the cochlea and for equilibrium they are in a number of canals collectively known as the endolymphatic system.

### A.4.1.2 For General Senses

In contrast to the special senses, the general senses refer to sensations distributed throughout the body. In general, standard texts describe five different kinds of general sensory receptors in the body: (1) thermoreceptors to feel hot and cold; (2) mechanoreceptors to sense light touch; (3) stereognostic receptors to understand the form and nature of objects by palpation; (4) proprioceptors to respond to position and movements of the musculoskeletal system; and (5) nociceptors to experience pain.

Quite a few histologic terms are used to describe receptors for the general senses, such as Merkel's disk, Meissner's corpuscle, paciniform ending, Vater–Pacini corpuscle, Rufini's corpuscle, Krause's end bulb, neuromuscular spindle, neurotendinous organ, tactile corpuscle, and free nerve ending. The roles of these structures are not understood, or is it understood if each of these structures responds to a unique type of sensation or if each is capable of responding to multiple types.

Because acupuncture is primarily concerned with nociception (the sense of pain), it is worthwhile to point out that the receptors for various pain sensations indicated by such adjectives as sharp, burning, dull, numbing, prickling, and tingling are also undistinguished. It is unsettled whether these different sensations arise from different receptors or combinations of receptors, or if they indicate different physiological reactions. It is settled that receptors for pain sensation are often described as free nerve endings with very little myelination, or "naked nerves." Consequently, nerve fibers for nociception are the smallest of all known nerves.[9] The mean diameter of these tiny nociceptor nerves, which are known as C fibers, is about 1 μm (1/1000 of a millimeter).

### A.4.2 EFFERENT FIBERS

Efferent fibers were briefly introduced earlier. The two kinds of efferent fibers are those to skeletal muscle and those to smooth and cardiac muscles.

#### A.4.2.1 To Skeletal Muscle

Skeletal muscles, except for those in the face and head, are innervated by efferent fibers to the skeletal muscles originating from motor nerve cells in the anterior horn of the spinal cord. The skeletal muscles in the face and head are classified as muscles (1) of mastication to control chewing movements of the mouth; and (2) of facial expression. The nerves that control the muscles of mastication are branches of the trigeminal (V) and arise from motor nerve cells located inside the brain in the motor nucleus of the trigeminal nerve. The nerve fibers that control facial expression are branches of the facial (VII) and arise from motor nerve cells also located inside the brain, in the motor nucleus of the facial nerve.

#### A.4.2.2 To Smooth and Cardiac Muscles

The cardiac muscles are those of the heart. The smooth muscles are found in blood vessels and all visceral organs and are often referred to as *involuntary muscles* because they are not typically thought of as being under conscious control. The innervations of smooth and cardiac muscles are referred to as *autonomic nerves* and, collectively, as the *autonomic nervous system.*

The autonomic nervous system is divided into the sympathetic and parasympathetic nervous systems, each consisting of two sets of neurons: preganglionic and postganglionic. Thus, there are four categories of autonomic nerve cells: (1) preganglionic sympathetic, (2) postganglionic sympathetic, (3) preganglionic parasympathetic, and (4) postganglionic parasympathetic. Preganglionic sympathetic nerves arise from preganglionic sympathetic nerve cells located in the lateral intermediate cell column of the thoracic and lumbar spinal cord; by means of their axons within the rami communicantes, they terminate in postganglionic sympathetic nerve cells housed in sympathetic ganglia situated along the side of the vertebral column (one of these ganglia is depicted in Figure A.2). From the sympathetic ganglia, the postganglionic sympathetic nerve fibers return through the rami communicantes to join the spinal nerves to distribute throughout the body. (In the thorax, the sympathetic ganglia from T5 through T11 are interconnected by the sympathetic chain.) When needles are inserted into the spinal nerves, the efferent postganglionic sympathetic fibers are among those stimulated.

In the parasympathetic nervous system, preganglionic nerve cells arise in the brain from structures known as the Edinger–Westphal nucleus and the superior and inferior salivatory nuclei. The structures that contain the postganglionic parasympathetic nerve cells are the ciliary, pterygopalatine, otic, and submandibular ganglia.

## A.5 NERVE BUNDLES

Nerve fibers congregate together to course through the body in *nerve bundles*, which are analogous to cables of electrical wire. These bundles typically consist of more than one type of fiber; they may be so small as to be invisible to the unaided eye. Larger bundles may be called *trunks* and assigned anatomical names. Often the terms *trunk* and *bundle* are used synonymously. The two main types of nerve bundles or trunks are muscular and cutaneous. Both types contain afferent sensory fibers and postganglionic sympathetic fibers to regulate the smooth muscle found in the walls of blood vessels in skin and muscle. The two types differ in that muscular bundles also contain efferent fibers to activate skeletal muscle. The cutaneous sensory fibers originate from sensory receptors in the deepest layers of the epidermis called the stratum germinativum and the stratum spinosum.

## REFERENCES

1. Pomeranz, B. Acupuncture and the endorphins. *Ethos* 10:385, 1982.
2. Pomeranz, B. and Chiu, D. Naloxone blocks acupuncture analgesia and causes hyperalgesia: endorphin is implicated. *Life Sci.* 19:1757, 1976.
3. Pomeranz, B. et al. Acupuncture reduces electrophysiological and behavioral responses to noxious stimuli: pituitary is implicated. *Exp. Neur.* 54:172, 1977.
4. Pomeranz, B. and Paley, D. Electroacupuncture hyperanalgesia is mediated by afferent nerve impulses: an electrophysiological study in mice. *Exp. Neur.* 66:398, 1979.
5. Pert, A. et al. Alterations in rat central nervous system endorphins following transauricular electroacupuncture. *Brain Res.* 224:83, 1981.

6. Wenhe, Z. and Yucun, S. Change in levels of monoamine neurotransmitters and their main metabolites of rat brain after electrical acupuncture treatment. *Int. J. Neur.* 15:147, 1981.

7. Wenhe, Z. et al. The effect of electric acupuncture treatment on urinary MHPG-sulphate excretion in unmedicated schizophrenics. *Int. J. Neur.* 14:179, 1981.

8. Ulett, G.A. and Han, S.P. *The Biology of Acupuncture.* Warren H. Green, Inc., St. Louis, 2002.

9. Bonica, J.J. *The Management of Pain,* 2nd Ed. Vol. I and II. Lea & Febiger, Philadelphia, 1990.

# Glossary

**Active phase:** the phase of an acupoint such that the point actively produces a sensation of pain without being palpated

**Acupoints:** loci on the skin which, when stimulated with needles, produce desired physiologic effects

**Acupressure:** a technique similar to acupuncture which involves stimulation of acupoints by applying manual pressure or pressure with a blunt device over the skin without actually piercing the skin

**Acupuncture:** (1) the insertion of fine needles into certain points on the skin for therapeutic purposes; (2) the stimulation of the nervous system with needles to affect its functioning

**Afferent nerve fibers:** nerve fibers that carry messages towards the CNS; dendrites

**Auriculopuncture:** acupuncture of the external ear

**Autonomic nerves:** innervations of smooth and cardiac muscles

**Autonomic nervous system:** the collection of autonomic nerves in the body, consisting of the sympathetic and parasympathetic nerves

**Axon:** a protoplasmic extension from the cell body of a nerve that carries information away from the cell body

**Basal joint:** the first carpometacarpal joint

**Central nervous system:** the brain and the spinal cord

**CNS:** central nervous system

**Conversion:** the process of changing phase from latent to passive, or from passive to active

**Cupping:** an affectation consisting of placing a warmed cup over the skin to draw out negative energy and "bad blood."

**Cutaneous nerve:** see "Cutaneous nerve bundle" below

**Cutaneous nerve bundle:** a nerve bundle containing afferent sensory fibers and postganglionic sympathetic fibers (contrast "Muscular nerve bundle" below)

**Cutaneovisceral reflex:** also called viscerocutaneous reflex; a reflex, mediated by splanchnic nerves, between visceral organs inside the body and acupoints on the surface of the body, such that changes in the visceral organs can be manifested as tender points on the exterior of the body, and that stimulating the exterior of the body can modify the functioning of internal organs.

**Dendrite:** a protoplasmic extension from the cell body of a nerve that carries information towards the cell body

**Dermatome:** the skin area innervated by a single spinal nerve

**Dorsal root ganglia:** ganglia for each of the 33 spinal nerves located just outside the spinal cord; also called "spinal ganglia"

**Efferent nerve fibers:** nerve fibers that carry messages away from the CNS; axons

**Electrical acupuncture:** placing an alternating current across pairs of needles, theoretically to increase stimulation

**Endogenous:** as applied to acupuncture, referring to systemic factors (including circulating neurotransmitters and possibly blood sugar fluctuations in diabetes and fluctuations in circulating thyroid hormones) that may cause acupoints to convert to the passive phase; may also refer to illnesses that cause pain (e.g. cancer)

**Exogenous:** as applied to acupuncture, factors outside the body that cause injury and pain (i.e. injuries)

**Fibromyalgia:** a misnomer for a condition in which most of the acupoints on a person's body are in the passive or active phase; it is the authors' hypothesis that this condition is actually a disease of the nervous system caused by excessive exposure to pain

**Ganglion:** the structure, found outside the CNS, which houses the cell bodies of bipolar neurons

**General senses:** afferent nerves for sensations distributed throughout the body: thermoreceptors, to feel hot and cold; mechanoreceptors, to sense light touch; stereognostic receptors, to understand the form and nature of objects by palpation; proprioceptors, to respond to position and movements of the musculoskeletal system; and nociceptors, to experience pain.

**Involuntary muscles:** cardiac muscle and the smooth muscles found in blood vessels and all visceral organs

**Latent phase:** the phase of an acupoint such that it is not tender to standard palpation pressure

**Laser acupuncture:** the stimulation of acupoints with a low-intensity laser beam

**Local conversion:** conversion of acupoints in a localized region of the body, usually in response to exogenous factors; also called regional

**Moxibustion:** acupuncture associated with burning materials tied to the end of the acupuncture needles, waved over the body, or placed directly on the skin (an affectation)

**Muscular nerve:** see "muscular nerve bundle" below

**Muscular nerve bundle:** a nerve bundle containing afferent sensory fibers, postganglionic sympathetic fibers and efferent fibers to activate skeletal muscle

**Myelin:** a sheath surrounding nerve fibers consisting of lipid (fat) formed by cells in the neuroglia

**Nerve:** a nerve fiber

**Nerve bundle:** a collection of nerves coursing through the body together and typically consisting of more than one type of nerve

**Nerve cell:** the structural unit of the nervous system

**Nerve fiber:** a portion of a nerve cell, or neuron, consisting of a dendrite or axon

**Neuroglia:** specialized connective or interstitial tissue surrounding nerve fibers and nerve cell bodies

**Neuromodulation:** the stimulation of the nervous system by whatever means to affect its functioning

**Neuromuscular attachment:** the site where a muscular nerve branch (consisting of motor, sensory and sympathetic fibers) attaches to and enters a muscle mass

**Neuron:** a nerve cell

**Neurovascular bundle:** nerves, arteries and veins coursing in close association

**Nociceptor:** nerve receptor for the sensation of pain

**Non-specific:** used to describe an acupoint that is passive in less than 25% of individuals and to describe an individual who has primary, secondary, tertiary and non-specific systemic acupoints in the passive phase (and who is often diagnosed with "fibromyalgia")

**Pain quantification:** 1) pain sensitivity; 2) the process of determining or estimating pain sensitivity by palpating representative points

**Pain sensitivity:** the approximate proportion of some 200+ acupoints on an individual's body that are sensitive to standard palpation pressure (i.e. in the passive phase), expressed on a 12-point scale, with zero being no passive acupoints and 12 being all acupoints in the passive phase

**Paravertebral points:** acupoints along the upper thoracic spine, from T2 to T6, thought to stimulate the sympathetic nervous system

**Passive phase:** the phase of an acupoint such that the examinee feels pain or aching with standard palpation pressure

**Peripheral nervous system:** all neural tissue or structure outside the brain and spinal cord

**PNS:** peripheral nervous system

**Postganglionic parasympathetic nerves:** nerves having their cell bodies in the ciliary, pterygopalatine, otic and submandibular ganglia

**Postganglionic sympathetic nerves:** nerves arising from the sympathetic ganglia and then joining the spinal nerves to distribute throughout the body

**Preganglionic parasympathetic nerves:** nerves arising in the brain from structures known as the Edinger-Westphal nucleus and the superior and inferior salivatory nuclei

**Preganglionic sympathetic nerves:** nerves arising from preganglionic sympathetic nerve cells located in the lateral intermediate cell column of the thoracic and lumbar spinal cord and terminating in postganglionic sympathetic nerve cells housed in sympathetic ganglia situated along the side of the vertebral column

**Primary:** used to describe an acupoint that is passive in more than 75% of individuals, or to describe an individual who has only primary systemic acupoints in the passive phase

**Pterygopalatine ganglion:** the ganglion of the facial nerve (Cranial Nerve VII)

**Randomized controlled trial:** a scientific study in which the subjects are randomly assigned to either treatment or control groups for comparison

**RCT:** randomized controlled trial

**Regional conversion:** local conversion

**Secondary:** used to describe an acupoint that is passive in 50-74% of individuals or to describe an individual who has only primary and secondary systemic acupoints in the passive phase

**Semilunar ganglion:** see "Trigeminal ganglion" below

**Sensory nerve fibers:** afferent nerve fibers (see above)

**Sets:** see "Treatment sets" below

**Special senses:** afferent nerves located in a special area, in the head, and each having a unique physiologic duty to perform; they are for smell, vision, taste, hearing and equilibrium

**Spinal ganglia:** see "Dorsal root ganglia" above

**Spinning:** a method of stimulating needles by gently rotating them between the thumb and index fingers

**Splanchnic:** visceral, or of the internal organs

**Standard palpation pressure:** two to three points of pressure per square centimeter, typically delivered by an examiner's fingertip

**Systemic conversion:** conversion of acupoints throughout the body in a generally predictable sequence, usually in response to exogenous factors

**Tertiary:** used to describe an acupoint that is passive in 25-49% of individuals or to describe an individual who has only primary, secondary and tertiary systemic acupoints in the passive phase

**Treatment sets:** three treatment sessions over the course of about a week, usually followed by a week's rest

**Trigeminal ganglion:** the ganglion of the trigeminal nerve (Cranial Nerve V); also called the "semilunar ganglion"

**Viscerocutaneous reflex :** also called cutaneovisceral reflex; a reflex, mediated by splanchnic nerves, between visceral organs inside the body and acupoints on the surface of the body, such that changes in the visceral organs can be manifested as tender points on the exterior of the body, and that stimulating the exterior of the body can modify the functioning of internal organs.

# Index